EDITED BY
BRIAN DOUCET, RIANNE VAN MELIK,
AND PIERRE FILION

VOLUME 1: COMMUNITY AND SOCIETY

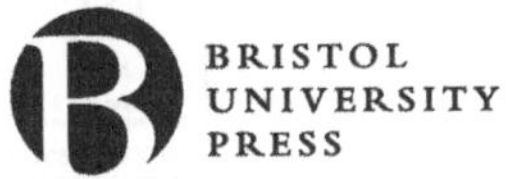

BRISTOL
UNIVERSITY
PRESS

First published in Great Britain in 2021 by

Bristol University Press
University of Bristol
1–9 Old Park Hill
Bristol
BS2 8BB
UK
t: +44 (0)117 954 5940
e: bup-info@bristol.ac.uk

Details of international sales and distribution partners are available at
bristoluniversitypress.co.uk

British Library Cataloguing in Publication Data
A catalogue record for this book is available from the British Library

ISBN 978-1-5292-1887-9 hardcover
ISBN 978-1-5292-1888-6 ePub
ISBN 978-1-5292-1889-3 ePdf

Cover design by blu inc, Bristol
Front cover image: FilippoBacci/istockphoto.com
Bristol University Press uses environmentally responsible print partners
Printed and bound in Great Britain by CPI Group (UK) Ltd,
Croydon, CR0 4YY

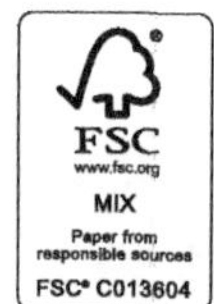

Contents

List of Figures and Tables

Figures

Tables

Notes on Contributors

Jeremy Auerbach is a postdoctoral Research Fellow in the Department of Environmental and Radiological Health Sciences at Colorado State University, US.

Nurul Azreen Azlan teaches in the MSc Sustainable Urban Design program at Universiti Teknologi, Malaysia.

Ajay Bailey is a Professor of Social Urban Transitions at the International Development Studies group, Department of Human Geography and Spatial Planning, Faculty of Geosciences, Utrecht University, the Netherlands.

Ellen Bal is an Associate Professor in the Department of Social and Cultural Anthropology, Vrije Universiteit Amsterdam, the Netherlands.

Niels Bartels is the Manager of Communications at the Leyden Academy on Vitality and Ageing, the Netherlands.

Nguyen N. Binh is a PhD candidate in the Department of Geography, McGill University, Canada.

Sheere Brooks is a Senior Lecturer and Researcher in the Faculty of Education and in the Faculty of Agriculture at the College of Agriculture Science and Education, Jamaica.

Higor Carvalho is a PhD candidate at the University of São Paulo, Brazil.

Diotima Chattoraj is a Research Assistant in the Department of Public Health at the National University of Singapore.

Jordin Clark is a PhD candidate within the Communication Studies program at Colorado State University, US.

Chrissie Cowan (Ngāti Kahungunu, Ngāti Porou) is the Chief Executive for Kāpō Māori Aotearoa New Zealand Inc., a national Indigenous organization founded by blind, low vision, vision impaired, and deafblind Māori and their whānau in New Zealand.

Jiska de Groot is a Researcher at University of Cape Town, South Africa.

Lieke de Kock is a Junior Researcher at Leyden Academy, the Netherlands.

Richardson Dilworth is a Professor of Politics and Head of the Department of Politics at Drexel University, US.

Brian Doucet is an Associate Professor and Canada Research Chair in the School of Planning at the University of Waterloo, Canada.

Sanjeeb Drong is Director of the Indigenous Peoples Development Services (IPDS) and General Secretary of the Bangladesh Indigenous Peoples Forum. He has been active as a human rights activist for nearly three decades.

Pierre Filion is a Professor in the School of Planning at the University of Waterloo, Canada.

Sobin George is an Assistant Professor at the Centre for Study of Social Change and Development (CSSCD), Institute for Social and Economic Change, India.

Ferhan Gezici is a Professor in the Urban and Regional Planning Department, Istanbul Technical University, Turkey.

Rebekah Graham (Pākehā) is based in the Waikato region of Aotearoa New Zealand and is a registered community psychologist. She also heads up Parents of Vision Impaired NZ.

Mallik Akram Hossain is a Professor in the Department of Geography and Environment at Jagannath University, Bangladesh.

Cansu İlhan is a Research Assistant and a PhD candidate in the Urban and Regional Planning Department, Istanbul Technical University, Turkey.

Beatriz Kara José is a Professor of Architecture and Urban Design at Centro Universitário SENAC, São Paulo, Brazil.

Charlotte Lemanski is a Reader in Urban Geography at University of Cambridge, UK.

Jolanda Lindenberg is a senior staff member and Researcher leading the focus area Connected at the Leyden Academy on Vitality and Ageing, the Netherlands.

Bridgette Masters-Awatere (Te Rarawa, Ngai Te Rangi, Tūwharetoa ki Kawerau) is the co-Director of the Māori & Psychology Research Unit (MPRU) at the School of Psychology, University of Waikato, New Zealand.

Olga Matveieva is an Associate Professor at Dnipropetrovsk Regional Institute for Public Administration of the National

Academy for Public Administration under the President of Ukraine.

Robin Mazumder is an environmental neuroscientist and recent PhD graduate from the University of Waterloo, Canada, who researches the psychological impacts of living in urban environments.

Solange Muñoz is an Assistant Professor in Geography at University of Tennessee, US.

Prajwal Nagesh is a doctoral student in the Department of Human Geography and Spatial Planning, Utrecht University, the Netherlands and Institute for Social and Economic Change, India.

Vasil Navumau is a Visiting Fellow at the Center for Advanced Internet Studies, Bochum, Germany.

Lorraine Nencel is an Associate Professor in the Department of Sociology, Vrije Universiteit Amsterdam, the Netherlands.

Sawyer Phinney is a PhD candidate in Geography at University of Manchester, UK.

Abdellatif Qamhaieh is an Associate Professor of Architecture and Urbanism at the American University in Dubai, UAE.

M. Feisal Rahman is a postdoctoral Researcher in the Department of Geography at Durham University, UK.

Roberto Rocco is an Associate Professor of Spatial Planning and Strategy at Delft University of Technology, the Netherlands.

Magdalena Rodekirchen is a PhD candidate in the Politics Department at University of Manchester, UK.

Luciana Royer is a Professor of Spatial Planning at University of São Paulo, Brazil.

Hanna A. Ruszczyk is an Urban Geographer in the Department of Geography at Durham University, UK.

Hosna J. Shewly is Senior Researcher in the Department of Social and Cultural Sciences, Fulda University of Applied Sciences, Germany.

Carolina Sternberg is an Associate Professor and Chair of the Department of Latin American and Latino Studies at DePaul University, Chicago, US.

Amanda Stevens is the Executive Officer for Deafblind Association NZ Charitable Trust, New Zealand.

Lekha Subaiya is an Assistant Professor at the Population Research Centre, Institute for Social and Economic Change, India.

Sarah Turner is a Professor in the Department of Geography, McGill University, Canada.

AKM Ahsan Ullah is an Associate Professor in the Department of Geography, Development and Environment at Universiti Brunei Darussalam, Brunei.

David van Bodegom is a Professor of Medicine in the Department of Public Health and Primary Care at Leiden University Medical Centre, the Netherlands, where he holds the Chair 'Vitality in an ageing population'.

Paul van de Vijver MD is a PhD student in Healthy Ageing at Leyden Academy on Vitality and Ageing and the Department of Public Health and Primary Care at Leiden University Medical Centre, the Netherlands.

Rianne van Melik is an Assistant Professor at the Institute for Management Research, Radboud University Nijmegen, the Netherlands.

Timothy P.R. Weaver is an Associate Professor of Political Science at the University at Albany, State University of New York, US.

Rose Wilkinson is Chief Executive for the Association of Blind Citizens of New Zealand Inc.

Sallie Yea is a Human Geographer at La Trobe University, Australia.

Acknowledgments

This volume is one of four in the Global Reflections on COVID-19 and Urban Inequalities series, edited by Brian Doucet, Rianne van Melik, and Pierre Filion. The editors of this series would like to thank Bristol University Press, in particular Emily Watt and Freya Trand, for their help and guidance while working with us to publish these books quickly. Thanks to Helen Flitton and Anna Paterson from Newgen Publishing UK for their detailed and timely work on copy-editing and production. We would like to thank the anonymous reviewers of our series proposal, as well as the individual manuscripts for their helpful and constructive feedback. We would especially like to thank Brayden Wilson, an MA student in Planning at the University of Waterloo, for his coordination of the administration of this project, including his frequent and thorough correspondence with over 70 contributors that helped to keep this project on schedule. Brayden's work was supported thanks to funding from Canada Research Chairs program, under award number 950-231821.

Territorial Land Acknowledgment – Brian Doucet and Pierre Filion work at the University of Waterloo and reside in the City of Kitchener, which are situated on the Haldimand Tract, land that was promised to the Haudenosaunee of the Six Nations of the Grand River, and is within the traditional territory of the Neutral, Anishinaabeg, and Haudenosaunee peoples.

Preface to All Four Volumes of Global Reflections on COVID-19 and Urban Inequalities

You are currently reading one of the four volumes of Global Reflections on COVID-19 and Urban Inequalities, which jointly explore schisms the pandemic has both revealed and widened, and measures taken to mitigate or eradicate these societal gaps. The aim of this series of edited volumes is to bring together a collection of critical urban voices across various disciplines, geographies, and perspectives in order to examine the urban challenges of COVID-19 and its impact on new and existing inequities in cities around the world.

There are two sides to the pandemic. As a highly contagious disease, given enough time and a lack of effective mitigation to restrain its spread, COVID-19 will eventually infect a large majority of the population, regardless of income or geography. This is why many public health measures are directed at entire national (or indeed global) populations. But we have also quickly learned that COVID-19 is selective in its effects – for instance, based on age and comorbidity – and that the pandemic and responses to it exacerbate fault lines traversing cities, societies, and, indeed, the world order.

There is a clear urban dimension to these inequities. Some parts of the city and some populations who reside in cities are more likely to contract and spread the virus. COVID-19 is thus an amplifier of pre-existing social divisions. Access to medical treatment and possibilities to physically isolate from potential infection are unevenly distributed. So too are the consequences of policy responses, such as lockdowns, the economic impacts of the pandemic, and the individual and political reactions it prompts. The pandemic has therefore increased divisions such as between young and old, rich and poor, left and right, and countless other societal dichotomies. As a result, experiences of urban life during the pandemic vary greatly. Where these impacts of the pandemic intersect with pre-existing racism, ageism, sexism, ableism, and spatial divisions within the city, the consequences have been particularly severe. As we write this preface, vaccines are starting to be produced, distributed, and administered. This poses new questions: will we emerge from the pandemic thanks to these vaccines? How equitable will the distribution of vaccines be within countries and at the global scale?

This context suggests myriad potential urban futures. The planning, policy, and political choices made in the short term will impact the medium- and long-term trajectories of cities and the lives of their residents. Moving forward, the challenge is how to ensure that planning and policy responses to the pandemic do not further exacerbate pre-existing inequalities and injustices that were amplified because of COVID-19. Therefore, there is a need for engaged, critical urban scholarship in order to ensure that issues of social justice and equity are front and center, not only in academic debates, but in rapidly evolving planning, policy, and public discussions that will shape these urban futures. Our four volumes suggest pathways that can help make this possible.

Rather than speculate, however, this book, and its three companions in our series, unites well-informed, reflective, and empirically grounded research from around the world to contextualize the new and amplified inequities brought about by COVID-19. The divisions that are apparent during the pandemic are not treated in isolation; they are firmly situated as part of long-term trends and broader narratives about cities, places, communities, and spaces.

Critical urban research during the pandemic

The first accounts of the novel coronavirus that would become known as COVID-19 emerged late in 2019 in Wuhan, China. Over the first months of 2020, the virus spread around the world. On March 11, 2020, the World Health Organization declared a global pandemic. Schools and businesses closed, office workers were told to work from home, and public spaces were shut. International travel came to a virtual standstill. Varying degrees of lockdown restricted the movements of people outside of their homes. In public, keeping distance from others and wearing facemasks became the norm. While the exact timing of these measures varied by country, by the summer of 2020, the majority of the world's population had experienced most of them. While the lockdowns did 'flatten the contagion curve', as restrictions of movement and activities were lifted, after a period of relative stability, infection rates took off again in the fall of 2020 and into 2021, reaching levels much higher than those experienced during the first wave.

As academics, we transitioned our own work during this time by setting up home offices, switching our teaching to online platforms, and adapting our research methodologies. The specifics of our own research shifted as it became impossible to study contemporary cities without assessing the impact of COVID-19. The more we examined our own research, however, it became apparent that the key questions and approaches driving our work remained central to interpreting this new reality. The inequities we were already examining in housing, transportation, public space, metropolitan regions, and planning systems took on new dimensions because of the pandemic. But most of the inequalities that are so central and visible during the pandemic were themselves not new; they were building, in different ways, on the pre-existing inequalities of cities before COVID-19. It soon became clear that COVID-19 was exacerbating and amplifying existing socio-economic and spatial inequities, even more than it was creating entirely new ones.

The pace of change during the pandemic poses a particular dilemma for researchers, who usually benefit from sufficient time to reflect and analyze. On the one hand, jumping too quickly to conclusions leads one to speculate rather than reflect, 'opinionate' rather than research. Academics are not journalists and it is not our task to provide real-time accounts and assessment of change.

On the other hand, as critical urban scholars, we must contribute to the discussions about the myriad ways COVID-19 is reshaping urban spaces and the lives of their inhabitants. Critical voices are more important now than ever, especially since cities face such uncertain futures and the responses to the pandemic will shape cities and urban life for years to come. COVID-19 has created urban challenges unprecedented in our lifetime. The pandemic has torn back the curtain on uneven social, spatial, and racial processes of urbanization that were previously downplayed in mainstream planning and policy debates. They have rendered visible some of what was previously invisible.

This context also gives rise to new possibilities and ideas that were once at the fringes of urban debates, such as closing streets to cars, which have been put into practice in cities around the world. But again, critical scholarship and research is necessary in order to study to what extent these planning and policy responses to the pandemic play a role in impacting (and potentially augmenting) the inequalities and injustices that are central to cities in the 21st century.

In short, it is simply not possible for urban researchers to 'sit this one out' while the dust settles. While academics may prefer to conduct research after the fact, this may be years into the future and after many important decisions have long been made. The challenge is therefore to strike a delicate balance between a slower, contemplative, and reflective approach to scholarship, while still striving to influence broader, rapidly evolving debates. We believe that our approach to this edited series strikes the right tone between these two important approaches.

The development of this edited series

Specifically, this four-part collection emerged from a meeting between our editorial team – Brian Doucet, Rianne van Melik, and Pierre Filion – and Bristol University Press in April 2020, wherein we were asked to assemble a rapid response book dealing with cities and the COVID-19 pandemic. As an editorial team, our approach has been to balance the need to make active contributions to rapidly shifting debates, while also reflecting on the impact the pandemic was having on urban inequities. We decided that short chapters, highly accessible to a diverse audience of scholars, students, professionals, planners, and an informed public, would be most suitable. The short nature of these chapters means that they fall somewhere between a typical media piece and a full-length peer-reviewed article.

A broad call for chapters was launched in mid-June 2020. Throughout various listservs and on social media, we invited researchers to reflect on how COVID-19 has impacted new and existing inequalities in cities throughout the world. We welcomed chapters that dealt with any urban topic and featured perspectives and voices not always central to mainstream scholarly, planning, or policy debates, including some co-written by non-academic authors.

The response to our invitation was overwhelming. We received many more abstracts than containable in a single volume. After a rigorous evaluation of the abstracts, we invited selected researchers to write full chapters. Keeping the best of these chapters, we found ourselves with a sufficient number of chapters for four volumes. The volumes were organized around the four main themes dominating the submitted chapters.

Given the edited nature of the book, the global scale of its chapters, and the wide scope of its object of study, there are inevitable gaps in the coverage of events relating to the pandemic, the reactions it has prompted, and the impact of all of this on different social groups. Also, it has proven impossible to provide cases from all parts of the world. All the same, the volumes do offer broad perspectives on different aspects of COVID-19 and their manifestation in different countries and continents. One of our goals was to include scholars from a variety of career phases, including early career researchers and graduate students, and to welcome chapters written in partnership with non-academic colleagues, many of whom offer insightful perspectives of lived experiences during the pandemic.

Each of the four volumes deals with a separate theme: Volume 1 is centered on Community and Society; Volume 2 deals with Housing and Home; Volume 3 examines Public Space and Mobility; and Volume 4 focuses on Policy and Planning. Each volume can be read as a stand-alone book, with a coherent theme, structure, introduction, and conclusion. But when read together, these four volumes synthesize research that reflects on the different ways in which the COVID-19 pandemic is reshaping urban inequities. While we have divided the volumes thematically, it is becoming increasingly clear that issues of housing, land use, mobility, urban design, and economic development (issues long siloed in urban debates) all need to be part of the same conversation about contemporary and future urban challenges. This is particularly true if social justice, equity, and the right to the city are to be central to the conversation. Many chapters throughout the series therefore focus on how COVID-19 *intersects* with different forms of inequality and injustice.

The timing for this project is particularly important. We gave contributors the summer of 2020 to write their chapters. Chapters were put together, not in the heated uncertainty of those first few months, but rather during a period when initial reflection on the pandemic's first wave became possible. While some chapters rely on media reports or carefully reflect on the early days of COVID-19, others draw on important and insightful fieldwork carried out during the spring and summer of 2020.

Much will have changed between when the volumes were written and when the series is available on physical and virtual bookshelves. This edited series is not a journalistic account of the pandemic. Instead, these volumes are a collective account of the first months of the pandemic, assembled with the idea that the knowledge, voices, and perspectives found within these volumes are necessary to shaping responses to the pandemic. The chapters presented in these four volumes serve as essential documentation and analysis of how the pandemic initially manifested itself within cities around the world, cities that were already becoming more economically, socially, racially, and spatially unequal. Understanding the early phases of this global pandemic is essential to dealing with its next waves and planning for the post-pandemic period. Likewise, understanding the consequences of how the pandemic intersects with urban inequalities is necessary in order to create more equitable and socially just cities.

ONE

Introduction

Brian Doucet, Rianne van Melik, and Pierre Filion

Pandemic imagery and urban inequalities

This series of four books explores the relationship between the COVID-19 pandemic and a variety of inter-related economic, social, spatial, and racial inequalities that have come to characterize cities around the world in the twenty-first century. Each volume explores a different, yet connected topic within urban studies, geography, and planning. This volume examines divisions within urban communities and societies and discusses to what extent the pandemic has created new inequalities, or amplified existing ones?

During the first wave of lockdowns that quickly spread around the world, images of empty streets, stations, squares, highways, and markets presented a dramatic view of cities that constituted an immediate break from the pre-COVID-19 era. Often juxtaposed beside images of the same spaces in far busier times, these photographs were almost entirely devoid of people who were otherwise hunkered down in their houses. They gave the impression that everything had changed and that life as we knew it had come to a standstill. They also gave hope of a return to normality, as once-busy places waited patiently for life to return back to the way it was (see *The Guardian*, 2020).

These images were, however, an overly simplistic, one-dimensional representation of cities under lockdown. The reality, in most areas of urban life, was far more complex. Rather than everything changing, the first year of the COVID-19 pandemic has also demonstrated that much has remained the same: the inequalities that characterized cities before the pandemic have been central to understanding both the unequal impacts of the virus on urban communities and the different ways in which the city has been experienced during the pandemic. These inequalities have been amplified, and the power relations that govern cities and urban space have barely changed: those who had little influence in planning and policymaking before the pandemic continue to be absent from them. While much of the world's attention is now focused on inequalities, individuals and communities who have long suffered injustices, and discrimination have seen little justice during the pandemic. This is important to remember when viewing images of cities during lockdown. While the dominant visuals have been of empty spaces, many people still leave their homes each day to perform essential work that cannot be done at home.

Photographing empty public transit has been a major genre within pandemic urban photography. Transit was also one of the most affected sectors during the first waves of the pandemic (Gkiotsalitis and Cats, 2021a). It was not just visual imagery of empty buses, trains and stations that spoke to this impact; ridership plummeted as office workers quickly transitioned to working from home, students took classes online, government directives in many countries prevented people from traveling even a few kilometers from their homes, and tourism all but dried up. While there is little evidence to indicate that transit vehicles are major places where the virus spreads, especially with mask requirements, proper ventilation, and regular cleaning (see Jones et al, 2020), many people avoided using it for even essential journeys out of fear of contamination (De

Vos, 2020; Qiu et al, 2020). Around the world, ridership fell between 60 and 90 percent from pre-COVID-19 levels within the first few weeks of the pandemic (Gkiotsalitis and Cats, 2021a; Orro et al, 2020). In India and other countries, public transport services were suspended entirely during early phases of the pandemic (Nagesh et al, Chapter Seven) A study in the UK concluded that the pandemic had set back attitudes towards public transport by decades, with a majority of respondents indicating that their cars were more important than before the pandemic and responding that they would not use their cars less, even if public transport was improved (Topham, 2020). At the other end of the transportation spectrum, 2020 also saw unprecedented demand for cycling, with cities around the world implementing new bicycle lanes (Agyeman, 2020; Butler, 2020a; Doucet and Mazumder, 2020; Scott (Volume 3); Mayers (Volume 4). In addition to creating space for recreation and exercise, bike lanes were implemented to provide alternatives for people wanting to avoid using public transport (Alderman, 2020; Laker, 2020; Wray, 2020).

However, even during lockdowns, some transit routes remained busy. Crowding on buses went from being an annoyance to a public health problem. Several early studies noted that transit occupancy levels needed to be between 6.5 percent and 18 percent of capacity in order to maintain 1.5–2 meter distances between passengers on vehicles and platforms (Gkiotsalitis and Cats, 2021b; Krishnakumari and Cats, 2020). This was compounded in many cases because public transport agencies around the world reduced service levels very early on in the pandemic. For example, in April, 2020, Singapore reduced transit service by two thirds and, consequently, instances of crowding were immediately reported (Tan, 2020).

While transit ridership dramatically declined everywhere, the severity of these declines varied between, and, importantly, within cities. Toronto, Canada's largest city and home to the country's busiest public transit networks, is a good example of the uneven geographies of decreases in transit ridership, and how these variations relate to the region's economic, social, spatial, and racial inequalities. The regional commuter rail and bus network that primarily brings office workers into downtown Toronto saw a decrease of over 92 percent. The city's transit agency, the TTC, saw a less steep decline, with 2020 ridership down 57.2 percent overall (Doucet and Doucet, forthcoming). However, even in March, 2020, during the city's first shutdown, when non-essential workplaces were closed, crowding was an issue on some routes (Marshall, 2020). They all had a few things in common. First, they were bus lines; subways, and the city's network of downtown streetcars were comparatively uncrowded. Second, they ran through inner suburban neighborhoods at the outer fringes of the city of Toronto, which were constructed in the decades after 1945, where a growing percentage of the city's low-income and racialized residents now reside (Hulchanski, 2010; Walks, 2020). Third, they served sprawling industrial areas with warehouses, factories, and distribution centers where employees could not work from home. Like many cities, Toronto's downtown skyline of bank towers and luxury condominiums belies the fact that manufacturing is the region's second-largest economic sector, most of which is dispersed throughout the suburbs (Walks, 2015). Pictures of these buses also made the rounds on the internet (Spurr, 2020), however, they did not capture the public's imagination in the same way that images of the empty city did.

Toronto was not unique to these trends, Liu et al (2020) found that in the United States, transit demand was highest in neighborhoods with greater numbers of essential workers, African Americans, Hispanics, females, and people over 45 years old. Hu and Chen (2021) examined ridership data in Chicago and found that while overall ridership declined by 72.4 percent, this was greater in areas with office-based employment and neighborhoods with higher percentages of White, educated, and high-income individuals. Declines in ridership were smaller in areas with more jobs in the trade, transportation, and utility sectors, as well as neighborhoods with more COVID-19 cases and deaths.

With these differences and uneven geographies in mind, it is clear that one image alone is insufficient to visualize the variegated trajectories and experiences of cities, communities, and societies during the pandemic. Therefore, to begin this book, and our series on urban inequalities and the COVID-19 pandemic, we have selected two photographs, taken at different locations within the same large urban region, at roughly the same phase of the pandemic. One depicts the lockdown city of privileged imagination: a previously busy downtown street that is virtually empty. This is juxtaposed with another image of a non-descript, ordinary industrial building, its parking lot full of cars. Both depict urban spaces without people. But in the second image, the cars remind us that many people leave their houses each day to go to work (see Gezici and İlhan, Chapter Six). While pictures reveal a lot about cities and urban life, they do not tell us everything, and therefore contextualization is required to help interpret them (Wyly, 2010). What this image does not show is that these workers are not entitled to any paid sick leave should they develop symptoms of the virus (or contract COVID-19 themselves), further amplifying differences in working conditions between different groups within the city. In early 2021, workplaces such as these were some of the biggest sources of outbreaks in Canada. There are, of course, many other important images of the pandemic city (see Arnold, Volume 3), but these two images are visual representations of the uneven geographies and experiences of the COVID-19 pandemic and how it has impacted people, communities, and places in different ways.

The main focus of the volumes within this series is to better understand how these uneven geographies of the pandemic intersect with pre-existing economic, social, spatial, and racial inequalities in cities around the world. Rather than speculating on future directions for cities, our emphasis is

Figure 1.1: Two views of the 'lockdown city', April 2020

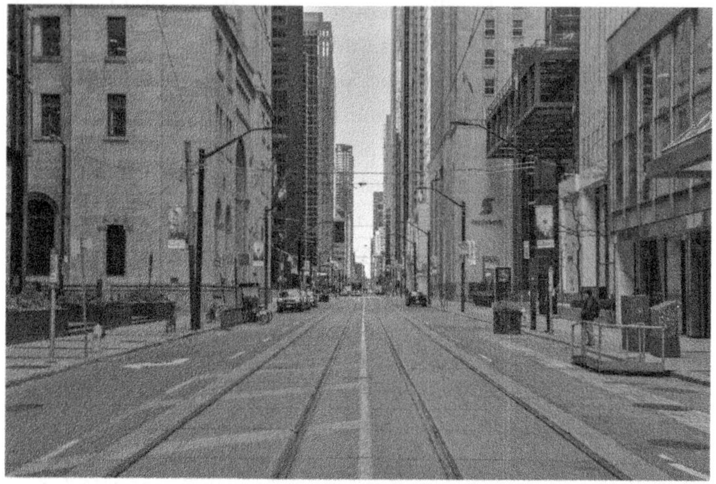

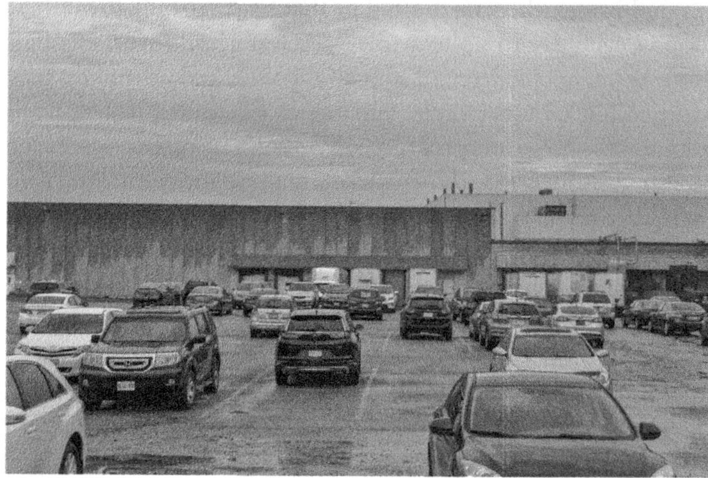

Source: Brian Doucet

critically analyzing and reflecting on what has changed, what has remained the same, and what conditions are necessary in order to shape a more equitable and just urban future. To do this, many chapters engage directly with marginalized communities, root their struggles during COVID-19 within longer trajectories of injustice, listen to their experiences of the pandemic, and use this knowledge to chart socially-just pathways to move forward into the post-pandemic period. This is important because the voices of those with lived experiences of poverty, discrimination, and marginalization are rarely front and center in planning, policy, and political debates that make and shape cities. Thus far into the pandemic, there are very few indicators to suggest that these power relations have changed.

Intersectionality and the pandemic city

Our experiences of the city are dependent on our gender, race, class, age, ability, and sexual orientation (see Mazumder, Chapter Seventeen; Lindenberg et al, Chapter Nineteen; Rodekirchen and Phinney, Chapter Twenty; Graham et al, Chapter Twenty-One). Geography also plays a role in this, with gentrification reshaping urban neighborhoods and poverty increasingly pushed to the spatial and social peripheries of the city. However, prior to the pandemic, these fault lines were often hidden, particularly within mainstream planning and policy debates (see Volume 4). The pandemic has rendered visible many of these pre-existing inequalities, particularly in public discourses. Therefore much of the critical scholarship on the impact of the pandemic in both the Global North and the Global South emphasizes how pre-existing inequalities (and the racism and discrimination that fuels them) have intersected with the pandemic to amplify already-existing social and spatial disparities.

As a result, the ways we have experienced the pandemic, and the impact it has on us, depends greatly on who we are and where we live. An intersectional lens that centers these differences is therefore a useful starting point. The term *intersectionality* was first coined by Kimberlé Crenshaw (1991), Professor of Law at Columbia University. She used it to describe how people's social identities can overlap. In a recent interview, she stated that intersectionality is:

> a lens, a prism, for seeing the way in which various forms of inequality often operate together and exacerbate each other. We tend to talk about race inequality as separate from inequality based on gender, class, sexuality, or immigrant status. What's often missing is how some people are subject to all of these, and the experience is not just the sum of its parts. (As quoted in Steinmetz, 2020)

In a similar vein, it is increasingly clear that topics such as housing, transportation, land use, racism, discrimination, economic development, and sustainability are highly related to each other and therefore cannot be treated as isolated conversations. While it may be easy for planners or policy makers to focus on a single issue, such as building a bike lane, this is not how many of the world's marginalized or racialized communities see, or experience, the city. Cycling advocate and planner Tamika Butler emphasizes this with a quote from Audre Lorde: 'There is no such thing as a single-issue struggle because we don't lead single-issue lives' (Butler, 2020a; 2020b). In a similar vein, Destiny Thomas (2020) also explicitly links transportation planning and racism when she states: 'if you want to ban cars, start by banning racism'.

Thinking about the Toronto example at the outset of this chapter, many pre-existing inequalities and injustices have been amplified during the pandemic. While 52 percent of the population self-identifies as being a member of a 'visible minority', by July 2020, 83 percent of the reported cases of COVID-19 were among non-Whites.[1] The city's White population saw only 17 percent of reported cases, despite constituting 48 percent of the city's population. The city's Black population was particularly affected by the virus, accounting for 21 percent of all cases, while comprising only 9 percent of the population (Cheung, 2020). Spatial disparities were also clearly evident. During the early days of the pandemic, infection rates rose at roughly the same level in the city's wealthiest and poorest neighborhoods. However, after the provincial government ordered all non-essential workplaces to close on 23 March 2020, the curve quickly flattened in the city's wealthiest and Whitest neighborhoods, predominantly found in the gentrified inner-city, or along subway lines. In its inner suburbs and other areas where low-income and racialized populations reside, infection rates kept rising and peaked almost two months later (Allen et al, 2020). It is important to note that the city's densest neighborhoods include areas with both the highest and lowest rates of infection, reflecting the polarized nature of gentrified condominium towers downtown that sit in stark contrast to aging apartment complexes in the suburbs that predominantly house low-income residents and new Canadians. These disparities continued into the first phases of the vaccine rollout, when the provincial government partnered with pharmacies to administer the vaccine. In the neighborhoods with the top five highest rates of infection (all inner-suburban areas in the city's northwest), no pharmacies were selected to take part. Pharmacies administering the vaccine were predominantly in the urban core where, conversely, infection rates have been very low. In the five neighborhoods with the lowest rates of infection (wealthy areas all in the city's urban core), a total of 12 pharmacies were administering vaccines (Roy, 2021).

Outline and structure of this volume

This volume is divided into four parts, and the chapters within them work to bridge the various siloed conversations that have dominated urban debates. It is important to note that much of the research featured within these chapters was conducted within the first phases of the pandemic, in early to mid-2020. The analysis, documentation, and reflection presented within these chapters are essential for understanding what happened early in the pandemic, in particular in identifying what changed, and, equally important, what did not. This detailed knowledge will remain critical for scholars, planners, and policy makers well into the future.

The first section of this book is on working practices, and begins with Sarah Turner and Nguyen Binh's chapter that takes an intersectional approach to examining experiences of migrant street vendors in Hanoi. They emphasize how pre-existing conditions of migration status, low-income, and informal working arrangements amplified the challenge of maintaining livelihoods during the pandemic. These conditions are also the main theme of Abdellatif Qamhaieh's study of migrant delivery workers in Dubai, featured in Chapter Three. Predominantly male and from the Indian subcontinent, these laborers perform tasks that others do not want to do. During the pandemic, they also put their own health at risk in order to make a living and keep much-needed supplies, such as food, delivered to more affluent residents who are able to remain at home.

In Chapter Four, Carolina Sternberg analyzes the working conditions of domestic workers (cleaners, nannies, caregivers) in the United States. Despite being on the frontlines of the pandemic, they have not been recognized as essential workers. Sternberg provides a detailed overview of the demographics, wages, benefits, and poverty living conditions of this group of workers, that constitute over 2 million people, 91.5 percent of whom are women. Sheere Brooks continues the theme of augmented precarity during the pandemic in Chapter Five. Brooks examines 'hustling' in Jamaica – a common practice of marginalized populations to capitalize on opportunities to earn an income in extreme economic landscapes. In Jamaica, hustling is a mobile, iterant, and unregulated activity that often involves street vending, or picking up side jobs; the pandemic has severely curtailed opportunities to earn income through hustling. This section concludes with a contribution by Ferhan Gezici and Cansu İlhan (Chapter Six), who provide an analysis of their study of who can work from home in Istanbul. They examine the employment sectors and residential neighborhoods where working from home has become common. Their findings echo studies from other countries and demonstrate that better-educated and higher-income individuals work from home at higher rates than lower-income and lower-educated individuals.

Part II of this volume is centered on life during lockdown, with chapters emphasizing how these experiences vary greatly between groups within the same cities, or how the lockdown rendered visible and amplified pre-existing inequalities and uneven geographies. In Chapter Seven, Prajwal Nagesh, Ajay Bailey, Sobin George, and Lekha Subaiya examine the impact of public transport restrictions on older adults in India. They deconstruct the idea that older adults are a homogenous group before exploring how reductions in public transit intersect with economic insecurity, isolation, and lockdown to amplify age-based inequalities. In Chapter Eight, M. Feisal Rahman and Hanna Ruszczyk discuss how the pandemic has exposed fault lines in food systems in a small city in Bangladesh. They identify specific challenges in smaller cities that lack the resources of larger ones to deal with challenges such as a pandemic. Their rapid-response research during the first wave of the pandemic builds on a larger project that was already examining food security and inequalities. Olga Matveieva and Vasil Navumau examine how government responses to the pandemic have exacerbated gender inequalities in Minsk and Kyiv in Chapter Nine. They explain that the contrasting experiences of the pandemic between the two cities is partly due to the vastly different responses and attitudes towards the virus in Ukraine and Belarus. They also note how, in both countries, life during the pandemic has been particularly challenging for women, albeit for different reasons. In Chapter Ten, Charlotte Lemanski and Jiska de Groot use the example of South Africa to highlight how the pandemic has exacerbated pre-existing inequalities with regard to access to health and other forms of infrastructure. They articulate that the ability to follow public health advice (which primarily stems from wealthy countries in the Global North) is privileged and that this advice requires local contextualization, particularly in the Global South.

Part II ends with a pair of chapters that provide intimate details on life during the pandemic. In Chapter Eleven, Jeremy Auerbach, Jordin Clark, and Solange Muñoz examine how the pandemic exposed existing gaps within larger systems and urban life, with a specific examination of how residents of a public housing project reimagined their lives during early phases of the pandemic. Their example in Denver demonstrates structural shortcomings, but also everyday community practices that emerged and point towards pathways for renewed stability and the reimagining of a more equitable society. Finally, in Chapter Twelve, Roberto Rocco, Beatriz Kara José, Higor Carvalho, and Luciana Royer profile the highly unequal lives of three Paulistanos (inhabitants of São Paulo) as they navigate new and existing challenges during the first wave of the pandemic. Their chapter sets out the structural circumstances that contributed to the city being a major pandemic hotspot and how the city's pre-existing economic, spatial, social, and racial inequalities are central to understanding how the virus has impacted different communities within Brazil's largest city.

Migration is the theme of Part III. It begins with Chapter Thirteen, written by Ellen Bal, Lorraine Nencel, Hosna J. Shewly, and Sanjeeb Drong, who examine the lives of young female migrants in Bangladesh, primarily employed in the ready-made garment industry, or in beauty parlors. They use the concept of liminality: a period of fundamental uncertainty characterized by a reversal or dissolution of existing social hierarchies where futures once taken for granted are cast into doubt (see also Banerjee and Das, Volume 2). In Chapter Fourteen, Nurul Azreen Azlan looks at the living conditions of migrants in Kuala Lumpur. She focuses on the overcrowded conditions that migrants have to endure, especially if they reside in city centers close to jobs, and equates contemporary responses to the pandemic among middle-class Malaysians to colonial European attitudes towards indigenous subjects.

In Chapter Fifteen, Diotima Chattoraj, AKM Ahsan Ullah, and Mallik Akram Hossain focus on life in a Rohingya refugee camp in Bangladesh, where experiences of social exclusion and 'Othering' have increased due to the pandemic. This exclusion is due to a combination of extreme health challenges, crowding, and a dramatic loss of economic livelihoods due to restrictions placed on interactions between those in the camp and those outside. Part III ends with Sallie Yea's chapter (Sixteen) which reflects on the outbreaks of COVID-19 among migrant workers in Singapore. In the first phases of the pandemic, these cases constituted the vast majority of infections in Singapore, which Yea's research attributes to a pre-existing political economy that both spatially contains and socially marginalizes migrant workers, and attitudes that see them as a risk *to* society.

Part IV focuses on different experiences based around age, race, gender, and ability. In Chapter Seventeen, Robin Mazumder articulates the concept of 'experiential equity' to explain how urban space is experienced differently depending on one's intersecting social identities. He relates this to the pandemic by reflecting on different experiences of cycling and asks who is able to fully enjoy new bike lanes that have sprung up in cities during the pandemic? In Chapter Eighteen, Richardson Dilworth and Timothy P.R. Weaver strike a hopeful tone when they argue that the profound instability and disruption that has been brought about because of the pandemic has established conditions for the 'defund the police' idea to shift from the margins of political debate into the mainstream. Jolanda Lindenberg, Paul van de Vijver, Lieke de Kock, David van Bodegom, and Niels Bartels discuss ageism and experiences of older adults in the Netherlands in Chapter Nineteen. Their work seeks to empower, elevate, and amplify the voices and experiences of older adults through the production of the website wijencorona.nl (Us and Corona), which collected the stories of older adults during the first few months of the pandemic.

Magdalena Rodekirchen and Sawyer Phinney argue in Chapter Twenty that, in the UK, pre-existing conditions such as austerity cuts to public services have disproportionately affected trans★ people, particularly through the loss of social infrastructure. This, in turn, impacts health, community, and housing. Finally, in Chapter Twenty-One, Rebekah Graham, Bridgette Masters-Awatere, Chrissie Cowan, Amanda Stevens and Rose Wilkinson examine how digital, as well as urban spaces, excluded blind, deafblind, low vision, and vision impaired (BLV) persons during the initial lockdown in New Zealand. Their intersectional chapter focuses on how New Zealanders with disabilities and/or Māori are over-represented within this digital exclusion. They find that the spaces inhabited during the lockdown prioritize the needs of a fully able citizenry. Volume 1 ends with a short conclusion where we question the idea that inequalities rendered visible during the pandemic will be reduced as the pandemic subsides, and articulate why power relations which govern cities will need to change if urban spaces are to become more equitable in the post-pandemic era.

Note

[1] Toronto is one of the few cities that keeps race-based data on COVID-19 infections.

References

Agyeman, J. (2020) 'Poor and black "invisible cyclists" need to be part of post-pandemic transport planning too'. *The Conversation*, May 27.

Alderman, L. (2020) '"Corona cycleways" become the new post-confinement commute'. *The New York Times*, June 12.

Allen, K., Yang, J., Mendleson R. and Bailey A. (2020) 'Lockdown worked for the rich, but not for the poor: the untold story of how COVID-19 spread across Toronto, in 7 graphics'. *The Toronto Star*, August 2.

Butler, T. (2020a) 'Why we must talk about race when we talk about bikes'. *bicycling.com*, June 9. www.bicycling.com/culture/a32783551/cycling-talk-fight-racism/

Butler, T. (2020b) *LiveMove Speaker Series: The Intersection of Racism and Transportation*. October 31. www.tamikabutler.com/media/2020/10/31/livemove-speaker-series-the-intersection-of-racism-and-transportation

Cheung, J. (2020) 'Black people and other people of color make up 83% of reported COVID-19 cases in Toronto'. *CBC News*, July 30.

Crenshaw, K. (1991) 'Mapping the margins: intersectionality, identity politics, and violence against women of color'. *Stanford Law Review*, 43(6): 1241–99.

De Vos, J. (2020) 'The effect of COVID-19 and subsequent social distancing on travel behavior'. *Transportation Research Interdisciplinary Perspectives*, 5: 1–3.

Doucet, B. and Doucet, M. (forthcoming) *Streetcars and the Shifting Geographies of Toronto: A Visual Analysis of Change.* Toronto: University of Toronto Press.

Doucet, B. and Mazumder, R. (2020) 'COVID-19 cyclists: expanding bike lane network can lead to more inclusive cities'. *The Conversation*, 22 November. https://theconversation.com/covid-19-cyclists-expanding-bike-lane-network-can-lead-to-more-inclusive-cities-144343

Gkiotsalitis, K. and Cats, O. (2021a) 'Public transport planning adaption under the COVID-19 pandemic crisis: literature review of research needs and directions'. *Transport Reviews*, 41(3): 374–92.

Gkiotsalitis, K. and Cats, O. (2021b) 'Optimal frequency setting of metro services in the age of COVID-19 distancing measures'. *Transportmetrica A: Transport Science*, DOI: 10.1080/23249935.2021.1896593

Hu, S. and Chen, P. (2021) 'Who left riding transit? Examining socio-economic disparities in the impact of COVID-19 on ridership'. *Transportation Research Part D: Transport and Environment*, 90: 1–14.

Hulchanski, D. (2010) *The Three Cities Within Toronto: Income Polarisation among Toronto Neighbourhoods, 1970–2005.* Toronto: Cities Centre Research Bulletin 41.

Jones, N.R., Qureshi, Z.U., Temple, R.J., Larwood, J.P., Greenhalgh, T. and Bourouiba, L. (2020) 'Two metres or one: what is the evidence for physical distancing in covid-19?' *BMJ*, 370: 1–6.

Krishnakumari, P. and Cats, O. (2020) 'Virus spreading in public transport networks: the alarming consequences of the business as usual scenario'. Delft: TU Delft. www.tudelft.nl/en/2020/citg/virus-spreading-in-public-transport-networks-the-alarming-consequences-of-the-business-as-usual-scenario

Laker, L. (2020) 'Milan announces ambitious scheme to reduce car use after lockdown'. *The Guardian*, April 21.

Liu, L., Miller, H.J. and Scheff, J. (2020) 'The impacts of COVID-19 pandemic on public transit demand in the United States'. *Plos One*, 15(11): e0242476.

Marshall, S. (2020) 'Mapping TTC crowding during a pandemic'. *Spacing Toronto*, April 1. http://spacing.ca/toronto/2020/04/01/marhsall-mapping-ttc-crowding-during-a-pandemic/

Orro, A., Novales, M., Monteagudo, Á., Pérez-López, J.B. and Bugarín, M.R. (2020) 'Impact on city bus transit services of the COVID–19 lockdown and return to the new normal: the case of A Coruña (Spain)'. *Sustainability*, DOI: 10.3390/su12177206

Qiu, J., Shen, B., Zhao, M., Wang, Z., Xie, B. and Xu, Y. (2020) 'A nationwide survey of psychological distress among Chinese people in the COVID-19 epidemic: implications and policy recommendations'. *General Psychiatry*, DOI: 10.1136/gpsych-2020-100213

Roy, I. (2021) 'Plenty of pharmacies, but no vaccines in Toronto's Northwest'. *The Local*, 25 March. https://thelocal.to/plenty-of-pharmacies-but-no-vaccines-in-torontos-northwest/

Spurr, B. (2020) 'Some Toronto bus routes still crowded despite COVID-19: what about social distancing?' *The Toronto Star*, March 27.

Steinmetz, K. (2020) 'She coined the term "intersectionality" over 30 years ago: here's what it means to her today'. *Time Magazine*, February 20.

Tan, C. (2020) 'Coronavirus: reduced frequency of trains leads to crowding on some'. *The Straits Times*, April 19.

The Guardian (2020) 'US cities in coronavirus quarantine, seen from above – in pictures'. *The Guardian*, March 23.

Thomas, D. (2020) ' "Safe streets" are not safe for Black lives'. *Bloomberg CityLab*, June 8.

Topham, G. (2020) 'Covid set back attitudes to public transport by two decades, says RAC'. *The Guardian*, November 9.

Walks, A. (2015) 'Stopping the "war on the car": neoliberalism, Fordism, and the politics of automobility in Toronto'. *Mobilities*, 10(3): 402–22.

Walks, A. (2020) 'Inequality and neighbourhood change in the Greater Toronto region', in J. Grant, W. Walks and H. Ramos (eds) *Changing Neighbourhoods: Social and Spatial Polarization in Canadian Cities*. Vancouver: University of British Columbia Press, pp 79–99.

Wyly, E. (2010) 'Things pictures don't tell us: in search of Baltimore'. *City*, 14(5): 497–528.

Wray, S. (2020) 'Bogotá expands bike lanes to curb coronavirus spread'. *Smart City World*, March 18. www.smartcitiesworld. net/news/news/bogota-expands-bike-lanes-overnight-to-curb-coronavirus-spread-5127

PART I

Working Practices

TWO

Street Vendor Struggles: Maintaining a Livelihood Through the COVID-19 Lockdown in Hanoi, Vietnam

Sarah Turner and Nguyen N. Binh

Introduction

Vietnam's first COVID-19 case was confirmed on 22 January 2020, with a second wave taking hold from July 2020. The Vietnamese government's initial mitigation strategies included a mandatory quarantine for travelers from COVID-19-affected countries and a strong public health campaign (Ivic, 2020). On 19 March, after a rise in cases, Hanoi People's Committee advised all residents to self-isolate at home until the month's end (Reuters, 2020). This preceded a national lockdown from 1 to 23 April 2020 following Directive 16, which temporarily closed all but essential services, resulting in rapid unemployment increases in both formal and informal sectors (Trần Oanh, 2020).

One of the informal sector groups hit hard by the pandemic and Directive 16 was Hanoi's migrant street vendors (VOA News, 2020). Street vending supports thousands of households in Hanoi and the surrounding hinterland, with those involved – predominantly women – often being rural-to-urban migrants who lack the formal education skills to secure 'modern' urban employment. They are drawn to the city due to opportunities to contribute to their broader household livelihoods, especially to pay for farming inputs and children's school fees. Yet, prior to COVID-19, these street vendors were already facing tough conditions, with a 2008 street vending ban covering 62 streets and 48 public spaces in Hanoi's urban core, curtailing access to favorable trading sites (Turner and Schoenberger, 2012). Directive 16 then halted their work completely, at least in theory.

This chapter draws on semi-structured interviews with 31 street vendors in Hanoi completed between May and July 2020 as COVID-19 restrictions relating to the first wave were lifting and before the second wave hit. Twenty-seven of the respondents were migrant vendors, while four were long-term Hanoi residents. We focus predominantly on migrant vendors here, given their already precarious situation on the city's streets, with responses from long-term resident vendors used for comparisons. Of our respondents, 28 were women, representative of street vendors in Hanoi as a whole (and across Vietnam). Our findings are also underscored by long-term research with Hanoi street vendors since 1999. Conceptually, we take an intersectional approach to urban informal livelihoods and inequality, analyzing how the interlaced axes of migrant woman or man, low socio-economic class, and informal worker created specific inequalities and/or barriers for individuals attempting to maintain urban livelihoods during this pandemic. Media articles have repeatedly reported that this virus does not discriminate – 'we are all in the same boat' – yet our work quickly reveals that this paints a false illusion of equality during times of livelihood shocks and crisis.

Initial impacts

The majority of Hanoi's itinerant street vendors are women migrants who rely on bicycles, poles, or baskets to ply their wares. The minority are fixed-stall vendors, typically long-term residents, for whom vending is often a means to stay busy in retirement and supplement small pensions (Turner and Schoenberger, 2012; Jensen and Peppard, 2003). Despite some migrant vendors residing in Hanoi for over a decade, they are often ostracized by authorities and 'native residents' as 'uneducated country-people' and 'outsiders'. When COVID-19 hit, most fixed-stall vendors paused their trading, using their state pensions or support from family members if they were able to tide them over. A few continued selling in front of their houses, especially those deemed to provide essential food-items including meat and vegetables. In contrast, migrant street vendors revealed that the initial impacts from COVID-19 included rapidly rising financial burdens and social stigma.

Rising financial burdens for migrant vendors

Although many itinerant vendors left the city to seek refuge in their hometowns before the April 2020 lockdown began in Hanoi (detailed later on; see also Banerjee and Das, Volume 2), a small proportion remained and tried to make ends meet (Pham Nga and Phan Diep, 2020). During lockdown, itinerant street vendors could be observed searching for customers, thus violating the government directive unless selling meat or vegetables (Hoàng Vũ and Quang Minh, 2020). As one woman who continued to sell fruit noted:

> The *Công an* [public security officials][1] told me, 'You kind of people never follow the rules!' But I told him, 'It's not that I don't observe the rules, but since I've bought all these fruit, I have to sell them … My children don't want

me to be out here selling on the street either.' I always think that those policemen, with their power, always see us as worthless people.

Another vendor, who initially stopped vending, noted that she had no longer been able to afford to obey Directive 16, despite risking her health and facing prosecution:

> I restarted selling about two weeks before they lifted the lockdown. We ran out of money so I had no choice […] The first few days [during lockdown], I was very afraid of the police, afraid of getting caught or fined. But I had to ignore it and go ahead, I had to go out making money for us to eat. (Lan, sticky-rice seller)

Vendors also noted that they had to trade longer hours post-lockdown as fewer residents were on the city's streets and business was far slower. Huong, a fruit vendor explained: 'Usually, when it's easy to sell, I head home early, but this year I only go back when it's already very late. Now it's common that I only manage to sell everything around midnight.'

The financial burdens of lockdown, slow business post-lockdown, and the prospects of another lockdown were extremely stressful for the itinerant vendor we interviewed. Concerns over access to basic necessities such as food was a recurring theme, with Ha, a vendor from neighboring Vĩnh Phúc Province, emphasizing: 'I was worried that if the pandemic had continued […] if it was like in other countries, then we would die, *really*, die of hunger if people could not work.'

The main coping mechanism vendors initiated in response to reduced incomes was to cut back on expenses, including food and other essential items. Yen, a vendor selling clothes, explained:

> I already cut back a lot on our spending, like skipping breakfasts or eating the leftovers from the night before…

> It's difficult with money now, I have to save most of what
> I make for my kids; to pay their tuition. We're having
> only plain rice with salt and sesame now.

When these restrictions were inadequate, some sought loans from private money lenders, resulting in high interest rates and additional stress. Van, selling clothes itinerantly detailed: 'We had to borrow some money; others had to borrow from the black credit market. It's difficult to borrow from relatives, because everyone is equally poor, so many have to go to the black market.'

Social burden and stigma

As COVID-19 cases rose, the nature of migrant vendors' routines – being mobile and interacting with numerous people on a daily basis – caused them to be perceived by the public, media, and authorities as potential risks to public health. Media reports with titles such as 'COVID-19 transmission risks among street vendors and beggars in Hanoi' (VTV24, 2020) stoked these fears. Even after the initial lockdown was lifted, many found they were unable to sell enough to get by. As reported in the media, one vendor noted: 'Now, because of the disease people shoo me away like a plague when they see me' (Pham Nga and Phan Diep, 2020).

The situation was not necessarily better for vendors who returned to the countryside before the April lockdown. Linh, an itinerant vendor selling pineapples in Hanoi for four years reported: 'People at our hometown treated us differently because we came back from Hanoi, so they were afraid and avoided us.' If vendors had been renting accommodation in a 'hotspot' neighborhood, where a COVID-19 breakout had been reported, their situation was even more complex: 'Back at the village, we experienced outright discrimination. Because they heard we were back from Bạch Mai hospital [a COVID-19 hotspot], they treated us differently. They thought we'd already contracted the virus' (Mai, fruit vendor).

Rising inequalities

The onset of the pandemic and subsequent government regulations created new inequalities along two divisions; first, within Hanoi's itinerant vending population, and second, between vendors and other urban workers.

New inequalities within itinerant vending sector

Vendors noted that those who sold certain items fared better than others immediately prior to, during, and after the initial lockdown. While limited numbers of itinerant vendors stayed to vend during the lockdown period, those selling meat and vegetables could at least attempt to make a livelihood, compared to others selling 'non-essential items' who were chased and fined heavily by *Công an*. Yet, as noted earlier, social stigma and a general lack of street life made this period tough even for essential-goods sellers. Moreover, with a general rise in unemployment and uncertainty, Hanoi residents cut back on non-essential purchases leaving vendors selling fruit, flowers, clothes, and religious items in a particularly precarious situation. Flower vendor Hue explained: 'If there'd been no COVID, people would have attended more [religious] ceremonies, festivals, like usual at the beginning of the year. So they'd buy more flowers as offerings. But this year, religious events were banned so people didn't buy many flowers.' Not surprisingly, vendors who usually targeted tourists or who supplied tourist cafés also faced stagnant sales: 'If tourists were still around, cafés would buy more from me, pineapples, avocados – to make juice to serve their guests... Before, when the tourists were still around, I could also sell to the tourists, but now they're not here, so I lose lots of customers' (Linh, fruit vendor).

Further inequalities compared to other urban workforce sectors

To support those negatively impacted by the April lockdown, the Vietnamese government adopted Resolution 42, a VND62,000 billion stimulus package to provide financial support for those who lost their income, including '*lao động tự do*' or informal sector workers (Trần Oanh, 2020). To be eligible, individuals had to have official documents from both their current and origin places of residence, and proof of low or no income. These criteria made it extremely difficult for informal workers to gain financial support, as the majority had no labor contracts to provide proof of income and struggled to obtain city temporary residence certificates (Di Lâm, 2020). Such regulations resulted in cases such as that of Vinh Tuy Ward in Hanoi, where 4,000 workers were identified as requiring aid, but only 47 proved to be eligible. Moreover, street vendors selling food only qualified if they held a valid business registration and food safety certification; since few did, they were immediately disqualified from receiving aid (Lan Phuong and Tat Dinh, 2020).

Vendors were frustrated at not being able to claim financial support, yet many noted that due to long-standing corruption they were not surprised they were deemed ineligible. Lan, a sticky-rice vendor explained:

> We're lost with the procedure and paperwork. Even with proper temporary residence registration here in Hanoi, it mightn't be enough. Only when you know someone who can 'guide' you through this process [for a bribe] might you get something.

The media reported that in response to criticisms regarding the lack of support for informal workers, the government-sponsored Fatherland Front Committee organized provisions for poor households (Trần Oanh, 2020). Local philanthropists also set up 'rice ATMs' in Ho Chi Minh City and Hanoi to provide 24/7 access to food for those who are unable to provide for their families following the nationwide lockdown (Duong, 2020). However, only a few of our interviewees knew of these initiatives, and only two had accessed the 'rice ATMs'.

Conclusion

Globally, it is estimated that almost 1.6 billion informal economy workers have had their livelihoods severely impacted by pandemic lockdown measures (International Labour Organization (ILO), 2020; see also Brooks, Chapter 5). This has certainly been the case in Hanoi, and in other Asian cities, where we are also tracking developments. In Hanoi, itinerant vendors – both women and men – have experienced sharp income declines, with many reporting cuts of half to two thirds of their pre-pandemic incomes, placing them in impossible financial situations (Pham Nga and Phan Diep, 2020; interviews). Facing gloomy trading scenarios, new social stigmas, and rising inequalities, a number of vendors who initially returned to Hanoi post-lockdown eventually departed again for their hometowns, abandoning their vending livelihoods and losing the incomes this had provided for family expenses. Yet, others were more resilient and, at times, defiant of government restrictions (see Thai et al, Volume Three). As one fresh-fruit vendor noted, 'After all, they still have to allow us to make a living and to survive, right? There are still many poor people in Vietnam, so if they're strict with us all the time, how will we make a living? In Vietnam, it's impossible to get rid of street vendors like us.' Whether public support and demand for street vendor goods will continue in this new climate is uncertain. Yet, Hanoi's street vendors have been the target of numerous government restrictions in the past and still ply the city's streets. With their history of resilience and adaptability, one can only hope that this livelihood option remains available for those directly reliant upon it, not only in Hanoi, but across the Global South.

Note

1   The *Công an* or *Công an phường* enforce government regulations, including Directive 16 and the 2008 Street Vending Ban, at the smallest official spatial unit of urban administration, the ward (*phường*).

References

Di Lâm (2020) 'Vì sao tiêu chí chi trả tiền hỗ trợ làm khó lao động tự do giữa mùa dịch COVID-19?' ['Eligibility criteria for COVID-19 support cause more troubles for informal workers?'] *Người Lao Động*, May 16. https://nld.com.vn/ban-doc/vi-sao-tieu-chi-chi-tra-tien-ho-tro-lam-kho-lao-dong-tu-do-giua-mua-dich-covid-19-20200516124051443.htm

Duong, Y. (2020) ' "Rice ATM" feeds Vietnam's poor amid virus lockdown'. *The Guardian*, April 13. www.theguardian.pe.ca/news/world/rice-atm-feeds-vietnams-poor-amid-virus-lockdown-436725/

Hoàng Vũ and Quang Minh (2020) 'Hàng rong len lỏi góc phố Hà Nội, người mua người bán không khẩu trang' ['Street vendors plying the streets of Hanoi, buyers and sellers without masks']. *Lao Động*, April 15. https://laodong.vn/photo/hang-rong-len-loi-goc-pho-ha-noi-nguoi-mua-nguoi-ban-khong-khau-trang-798452.ldo

International Labour Organization (ILO) (2020) 'As job losses escalate, nearly half of global workforce at risk of losing livelihoods'. www.ilo.org/global/about-the-ilo/newsroom/news/WCMS_743036/lang--en/index.htm

Ivic, S. (2020) 'Vietnam's response to the COVID-19 outbreak'. *Asian Bioethics Review*, 12: 341–7.

Jensen, R. and Peppard, D.M. (2003) 'Hanoi's informal sector and the Vietnamese economy: a case study of roving street vendors'. *Journal of Asian and African Studies*, 38(1):71–84.

Lan Phuong and Tat Dinh (2020) 'Hanoi overlooks street vendors in Covid-19 incentive'. *VN Express*, June 23. https://e.vnexpress.net/news/news/hanoi-overlooks-street-vendors-in-covid-19-incentive-4119749.html

Pham Nga and Phan Diep (2020) 'Covid-19 outbreak puts the poor in dire straits'. *VN Express*, April 2. https://e.vnexpress.net/news/news/covid-19-outbreak-puts-the-poor-in-dire-straits-4078029.html

Reuters (2020) 'Vietnam to ease nationwide coronavirus lockdown'. *Bangkok Post*, April 22. www.bangkokpost.com/world/1905235/vietnam-to-ease-nationwide-coronavirus-lockdown

Trần Oanh (2020) 'Lao động tự do chật vật trong dịch COVID-19: không ai bị bỏ lại phía sau' ['Informal workers during COVID-19: no one is left behind']. *Kinh tế Đô thị*, April 18. http://kinhtedothi.vn/lao-dong-tu-do-chat-vat-trong-dich-covid-19-khong-ai-bi-bo-lai-phia-sau-381578.html

Turner, S. and Schoenberger, L. (2012) 'Street vendor livelihoods and everyday politics in Hanoi, Vietnam: the seeds of a diverse economy?' *Urban Studies*, 49(5):1027–44.

VOA News (2020) 'Vietnam's virus checkpoints screen for fevers, limit urban movement', April 14. www.voanews.com/science-health/coronavirus-outbreak/vietnams-virus-checkpoints-screen-fevers-limit-urban-movement

VTV24 (2020) 'Nguy cơ lây nhiễm COVID-19 từ người ăn xin, bán hàng rong ở Hà Nội' ['COVID-19 transmission risks among street beggars and vendors in Hanoi'], April 11. https://vtv.vn/chuyen-dong-24h/nguy-co-lay-nhiem-covid-19-tu-nguoi-an-xin-ban-hang-rong-o-ha-noi-20200411190153125.htm

THREE

The Man and the Scooter: How the Low-Income Worker Helps Save a Locked-Down City

Abdellatif Qamhaieh

Introduction

Within the Gulf Cooperation Council (GCC) countries, the fate of the low-income migratory worker has always been a contested issue (Ewers and Dicce, 2016). Large numbers of migrant workers, mainly originating from South Asian countries, represent an important demographic in the region. In Dubai, the focus of this chapter, the concept of home deliveries has become common in the last few years. Armed with a scooter (a small motorcycle), a vast army of these low-income workers delivers goods quickly to homes across the city. Smartphone-based apps and third-party delivery operators have made this phenomenon even more wide-spread in recent years (Johnson, 2014). It is common to see these small scooters maneuvering traffic continuously, with their numbers growing steadily.

Early in the COVID-19 pandemic, cities in the United Arab Emirates (UAE) went into a strict lockdown and near-curfew conditions. Residents stayed indoors, and society came to a complete halt, similar to other countries around the world. In addition to emergency services and the construction sector, delivery services were some of the few expected to continue working and serving the residents during the lockdown. The delivery scooters were suddenly the lifeline of the city. Drivers continued to deliver goods to the city's residents, despite the obvious concerns for their own health.

This chapter argues that the COVID-19 pandemic magnified existing socio-economic divides and put them on full display. Vulnerable migrant-laborers had no option but to continue working at a time of great uncertainty, especially since much was still unknown about the virus, how it spreads, and its potential treatments. Similar to other urban poor around the world, they bore the brunt of the virus in order to make a living (see Part III). This chapter sheds some light on migration and urban inequality in the Gulf. It then highlights the added pressures of the pandemic as it disproportionately impacts the lower-income segments within Dubai.

Urban inequality in the Gulf

The Gulf states have a long history with migration. Throughout the early history of the region, labor-flows from Iran and the Indian subcontinent were common. With the oil discoveries and the oil boom in the 1960s and 1970s, the drive to build and develop became instant. At the time, coastal sheikdoms such as UAE, Qatar, Bahrain, and Kuwait, had small native populations, so a large amount of labor was needed to build infrastructure and cities. A significant demographic shift took place due to what is considered to be the third-largest migratory flow in modern history (Gardner, 2010). Today, for example, roughly 90 percent of the UAE's population are expatriates, varying in skill-level and national background.

Migration into the Gulf region is unique in several ways. It rarely leads to permanent residency or nationalization (with the exception of Bahrain). All expatriates in the Gulf are considered to be temporary non-citizens or guest workers. They are expected to eventually return to their home countries. Furthermore, due to the proximity to the Indian subcontinent, large numbers of low-income, blue-collar workers in the GCC originate from that area specifically. Their presence in the region's cities is evident, as they represent a sizable majority of the expatriates (Mohammad and Sidaway, 2012).

The conditions of this low-income workforce in the Gulf have always been a subject of criticism, especially in academic literature. However, important steps have been taken in the last few years to improve their living and working circumstances. The demographics of this workforce is primarily young; South Asian males are customarily referred to as *bachelors*. Though some are married and have families back home, they still do not earn enough to meet the minimum requirements for sponsoring their families' residency visas – *hence the name* (Mohammad and Sidaway, 2012).

These *bachelors* constitute the urban poor within the region. They receive the lowest salaries and live a very rudimentary living, at least compared to other expatriates (Walsh, 2006). They send the majority of their income to their home countries in the form of remittances. Language barriers, education levels, working conditions, housing problems, and regulatory restrictions keep them excluded from mainstream society. They usually interact with the rest of the community only when performing a service – such as food delivery.

Dubai: the global city, the divided city

Dubai has emerged as a global hub over the last two decades. It is a brand that has become synonymous with luxury, and high-end ritzy living. As a city, Dubai has grown dramatically over the last three decades (Pacione, 2005; Bagaeen, 2007). Within a short period, it transformed from a small port-town into a glamorous city, home to nearly three million residents.

Artificial islands, spectacular infrastructure, and unique architectural masterpieces, including the world's tallest tower, have made Dubai *the* destination in the region for millions of tourists annually. Thousands of new jobseekers also arrive every year from around the world. It is a city famous for its nightlife, shopping malls, and beautiful beaches – an alluring oasis in a climatically harsh and politically unstable region.

Despite the glamour, Dubai is a divided city (Buckley, 2013). The gap between the haves and the have-nots is very distinct and visible. On one hand, the country's nationals and the professional Western and Arab expatriates enjoy relatively comfortable, if not glamourous, lifestyles (Walsh, 2006). Meanwhile, the low-income workers (that is, the *bachelors*) have a rather harsh existence. They live on the periphery of society, busy in a life of hard labor with only an outsider's view of the surrounding glamour. They represent a sizable population, yet a silent one. They provide valuable services to the community, without which it would not function. Still they remain casual observers, and are never really expected to belong or participate.

Delivery and workers

Delivery services are a significant convenience of life in Dubai. Nearly everything in the city can be delivered for free or with a very minimal fee to the end consumer. This is especially true within the food sector and the small retail and grocery sectors. These deliveries take place atop a small scooter (motorcycle) with a delivery box attached to its back (Figure 3.1). Motorcycle delivery is typical in several Asian countries (Pinch and Reimer, 2012), and is not native or unique to the UAE. During the last few years, app-based deliveries became very common. Food and grocery items are ordered and delivered online with convenience. Third-party apps assume the role of the middleman between the businesses and the consumers (see also Mezzadra et al, Volume Four).

Figure 3.1: Delivery scooters and drivers awaiting orders

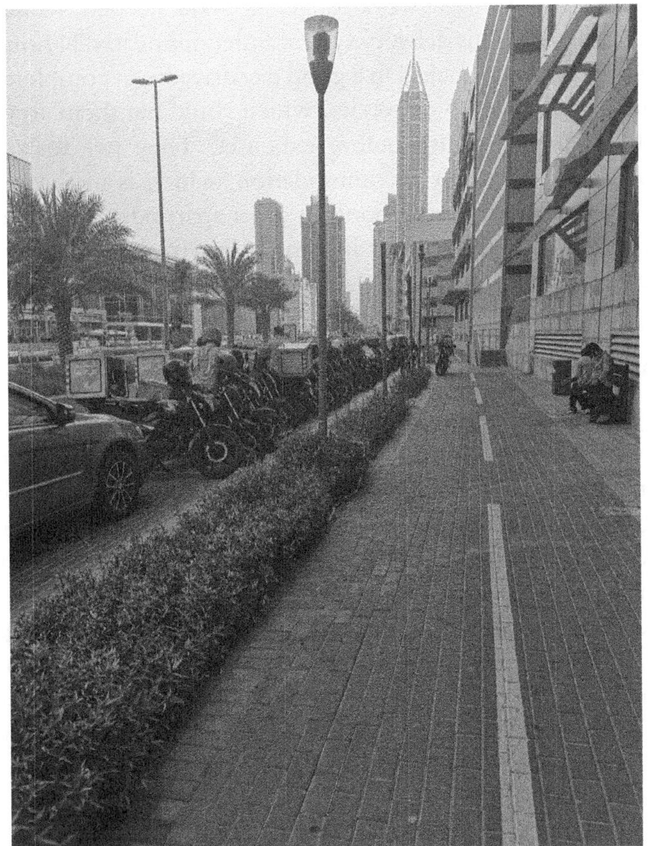

Source: author (August 18, 2020)

Motorcycles, typically driven by *bachelors*, handle these deliveries. They are often distributed in the city in different zones, waiting to receive instructions for pickup and distribution through their company provided cellphones (Johnson, 2014). They do not receive salaries but receive only a commission per delivery (10 AED or around 3 USD for each). The motorcycle is provided by their employer, whereas the driver pays for the gasoline. Their official working shift is eight hours, whereas some might work longer hours if needed, to make extra income. This delivery system functions nearly 24 hours a day, seven days a week. On a good day drivers can complete an average of ten to 15 deliveries, which could net them around 800 USD per month before expenses. They pay for their own food, and their accommodation, which is in the form of bedspace and shared rooms in older apartments. They also send the majority of their income home to their families in the form of remittances (Malecki and Ewers, 2007).

Early COVID-19 in Dubai

Arguably, the United Arab Emirates had one of the best global responses to COVID-19 during the first wave of the pandemic. Early on, government-imposed restrictions and rigorous enforcement of social distancing, disease tracking, and mask requirements spared the country from extensive community spread. Door-to-door testing, field hospitals, and testing roadblocks for cars kept cases at bay. As of August 2020, the country had around 65,000 cases, with approximately 58,000 recoveries and 330 recorded deaths (Ministry of Health and Prevention (MOHAP), 2020). This was despite the reopening of businesses and the return of limited tourism and flight services.

In the initial stages of the pandemic, and as Dubai started to deal with a growing number of cases, certain restrictions on movement were put in place, followed by a strict month-long lockdown. The lockdown began with a night-time curfew, then soon became a full 24-hour curfew. Residents could only go out for grocery shopping, but only after applying for an online permit associated with their car's license plate. Only one person was allowed per car, and some of the latest AI-driven traffic cameras and technologies were used to fine violators and made sure the lockdown was near complete. It was a strict yet successful operation and a testament to the efficiency of the response and the capability of the responsible government agencies.

During this period, only essential sectors were allowed to move around the city. These included emergency, medical, grocery, and delivery services. On the other hand, the construction sector was fully functional, despite the apparent dangers and with no official explanation for such a decision. There was no official breakdown of where and how infections were taking place. Significant infections appeared to be focused within the higher-density older areas, where most of the shared accommodations for *bachelors* are located (Badam, 2020).

Interviews

Six unstructured interviews were conducted with delivery drivers in August 2020, to understand their experience during the pandemic, especially during the full-lockdown period. All the drivers were of Pakistani origin and the interviews were conducted in English, though some of the respondents had difficulty expressing themselves and had limited English language skills.

The drivers indicated that their work increased during the lockdown due to the high demand for deliveries. They also discussed strict health measures and safety procedures mandated by their employers. These were further enforced by systematic corporate and police inspections. All were required to wear masks, gloves, and use sanitizers regularly. Some drivers complained that customers stopped paying much-needed and customary tips for fear of interacting with them. Many customers also opted for touchless delivery, in which drivers leave the goods or food outside, and the customers then pick them up after the driver leaves. Drivers expressed concerns about their health and noted that their families overseas were also concerned for their well-being. They were worried about interacting with people and potentially getting infected themselves. Some of them reported that customers often shouted at them or expressed anger, especially if the delivery mechanism or timing were not perfect.

Respondents expressed their initial desire to remain in their homes, especially during the total-lockdown period. Still, they indicated that they were not able to do so since they were paid by commission – so they would have no income otherwise. They also discussed their inadequate living arrangements, with many occupants per room in their shared accommodations. In their view, there was no possibility for social distancing, and they had a constant fear of infections. Still, they indicated that routine housing and health inspections by the authorities kept them safe. One of the respondents claimed that Pakistanis' don't get COVID-19! Though a small sample size due to the nature of this short study, these responses appeared to echo sentiments reported in media outlets related to delivery work during lockdown, as discussed by Zacharias (2020).

Conclusion

The conditions experienced by delivery drivers in the pandemic were essentially an extension of their difficult living and working conditions before it started, a trend noted by many chapters in this book. The crisis, though, sharpened the inequalities within the society and highlighted their plight even more. The more affluent segments of the city could enjoy the safety and isolation of their homes while receiving their daily needs – thanks to the delivery services. The vulnerable *bachelor*, though, could not afford such luxuries. On the one hand, he was expected, if not required, to work by his employers as there was an increased demand for deliveries. On the other hand, staying home to preserve his safety and health was not an option. He goes from house to house, risking infection himself, providing service for the community, albeit at the smallest of wages. As a low-income day laborer with no monthly salary, he needed the income and could not afford to take time off.

The crowded accommodations and living arrangements were also very problematic and made social distancing near impossible (see also Yea, Chapter 16).

However, attitudes from the rest of society highlighted a more significant problem: the disdain and negative views towards this population. Somewhat normalized, the negative attitudes towards *bachelors* were on full display in the city during these delivery 'transactions'. While drivers provided valuable services in such a critical period, the notion that they could be carrying and spreading the virus exacerbated the situation even more. Though the early COVID-19 response in Dubai was hailed as a success, already-vulnerable groups were being impacted more than the rest. Meanwhile, the pressures of the pandemic highlighted and sharpened societal flaws. City planners and policy makers need to address the source of some of these urban and social inequalities as they contribute to a divided society. Better working terms and conditions and housing improvements for this group should be the first of many necessary steps towards creating more equitable communities in the post-pandemic period.

References

Badam, R. (2020) 'Coronavirus: restrictions ease for residents of Dubai's locked down Al Ras district'. *The National*, April 28. www.thenational.ae/uae/health/coronavirus-restrictions-ease-for-residents-of-dubai-s-locked-down-al-ras-district-1.1011232

Bagaeen, S. (2007) 'Brand Dubai: the instant city, or the instantly recognizable city'. *International Planning Studies*, 12(2): 173–97. https://doi.org/10.1080/13563470701486372

Buckley, M. (2013) 'Locating neoliberalism in Dubai: migrant workers and class struggle in the autocratic city'. *Antipode*, 45(2): 256–74. https://doi.org/10.1111/j.1467-8330.2012.01002.x

Ewers, M.C. and Dicce, R. (2016) 'Expatriate labour markets in rapidly globalising cities: reproducing the migrant division of labour in Abu Dhabi and Dubai'. *Journal of Ethnic and Migration Studies*, 42(15): 2448–67. https://doi.org/10.1080/1369183X.2016.1175926

Gardner, A.M. (2010) *City of Strangers: Gulf Migration and the Indian Community in Bahrain*. Ithaca: ILR Press.

Johnson, S. (2014) 'Appetising apps to help you find good food'. *The National*, April 1. www.thenational.ae/lifestyle/food/appetising-apps-to-help-you-find-good-food-1.268006

Malecki, E.J. and Ewers, M.C. (2007) 'Labor migration to world cities: with a research agenda for the Arab Gulf'. *Progress in Human Geography*, 31(4): 467–84. https://doi.org/10.1177/0309132507079501

Ministry of Health and Prevention (MOHAP) (2020) 'COVID-19 information center – Ministry of Health and Prevention – UAE'. August 20. www.mohap.gov.ae/en/AwarenessCenter/Pages/COVID19-Information-Center.aspx

Mohammad, R. and Sidaway, J.D. (2012) 'Spectacular urbanization amidst variegated geographies of globalization: learning from Abu Dhabi's trajectory through the lives of South Asian men'. *International Journal of Urban and Regional Research*, 36(3): 606–27. https://doi.org/10.1111/j.1468-2427.2011.01099.x

Pacione, M. (2005) 'Dubai'. *Cities*, 22(3): 255–65. https://doi.org/10.1016/j.cities.2005.02.001

Pinch, P. and Reimer, S. (2012) 'Moto-mobilities: geographies of the motorcycle and motorcyclists'. *Mobilities*, 7(3): 439–57. https://doi.org/10.1080/17450101.2012.659466

Walsh, K. (2006) ' "Dad says I'm tied to a shooting star!" Grounding (research on) British expatriate belonging'. *Area*, 38(3): 268–78.

Zacharias, A. (2020) 'Coronavirus: Dubai's delivery drivers tell of life on the road as they count cost of Covid-19'. *The National*, April 5. www.thenational.ae/uae/health/coronavirus-dubai-s-delivery-drivers-tell-of-life-on-the-road-as-they-count-cost-of-covid-19-1.1000101

The Hidden Inequities and Divisions among Workers in the US: The Domestic Workers' Workforce as Non-Essential Workers

Carolina Sternberg

Introduction

The COVID-19 pandemic has laid bare the many ways in which domestic workers (housecleaners, nannies, and caregivers) remain undervalued, unprotected, and invisible across US cities. Over 2.2 million domestic workers in the US – 91.5 percent of whom are women – today face profound challenges and risks. As their employers take safety measures to practice social distancing, the so-called 'low-touch' economy has become widespread, and in April 2020 left 68 percent of domestic workers surveyed with no jobs according to the National Domestic Workers Alliance (NDWA) national survey (NDWA, 2020a).

At the same time, the vast majority of domestic workers are excluded from the protections of key federal labor laws and standards, including the right to minimum wage and those protections guaranteed under the Occupational Safety and Health Act (OSHA) and the Family Medical Leave Act. Currently, only ten US states and the city of Seattle have passed the Bill of Rights for Domestic Workers and yet, they lack Personal Protective Equipment (PPE) and are at the good disposition of employers who choose to pay them while they are not working. All these aspects combined constitute strong limitations for improving domestic workers' working conditions.

This chapter aims to provide an overview of the demographics, wages, benefits, and poverty living conditions of the domestic workers who, despite being on the frontlines of the pandemic, caring for the sick, and keeping homes clean, are yet not publicly recognized as essential workers. In addition, this work highlights the complex relationship between employer-employee and some of the incredible work that non-for-profit organizations across US cities have undertaken in order to improve domestic employees' working conditions and advocate for better workers' rights.

Key demographics on domestic workers and working conditions in the US

Feminists have long pointed to ways in which care work is privatized and devalued. Now we are witnessing an intensification of these processes in ways that affect us all deeply. Today, a disproportionate amount of care work is carried out by minority ethnic, immigrants, and women. Care work is itself 'systematically devalued as the feminized, private work of home, rather than as society's work' (Lawson, 2007: 2). The following study speaks volumes about how we need to start building new forms of relationships, institutions, and actions that enhance mutuality, well-being, and constructive engagement.

According to a recent study by the Economic Policy Institute on domestic workers in the US (Wolfe et al, 2020) those who care for our family members and clean our homes face long-term uncertainty, with 66 percent reporting that they are unsure if their clients will give them their jobs back after the pandemic. The decline in employment for domestic workers represents a significant loss of income for these workers and their families. The following are key and critical findings of this study (see Wolfe et al, 2020).

While women of all races and ethnicities are overrepresented (91.5 percent) in the domestic employee workforce, this over-representation is highly racialized with the highest share of Latinx workers (61.5 percent) employed as housecleaners. As for agency-based care workers, they constitute the domestic worker occupation with the highest share of Black, non-Latinx workers (30.3 percent).

This study also reveals that one third (35.1 percent) of domestic workers are foreign born, compared with 17.1 percent of other workers. One in five (20.3 percent) domestic workers is a noncitizen – housecleaners are the highest share in occupation – compared with 8.7 percent of workers in other occupations. Those noncitizens who are undocumented are particularly vulnerable in the workplace and are not eligible for unemployment benefits – one of the main sources of income for workers who have lost wages due to COVID-19 – even under the updated 2021 Coronavirus Aid, Relief, and Economic Security (CARES) Act.

In addition, there is a large and persistent wage gap between the median hourly wage of domestic workers – consistent across all occupations – and the median hourly wage of all other workers. Since 2012 when Burnham and Theodore (2012) released the first comprehensive report on domestic workers on 14 metropolitan cities across the US, these workers have seen stagnant wages. The average domestic worker is paid $12.01 per hour including overtime, tips, and commissions, 39.8 percent less than other types of workers (who are paid $19.97 per hour). Even when compared to similar workers, domestic workers on average are paid only 74 cents for every dollar that their peers make. These numbers also vary across races and ethnicities (see Burnham and Theodore, 2012).

As for poverty, the study notes that within the US, domestic workers are three times as likely to be living in poverty as other workers, and almost three times as likely to either be in poverty, or be above the poverty line and without sufficient income to make ends meet. Fewer than one in ten domestic workers receive some benefits through an employer-provided retirement plan and just one in five receives health insurance coverage through their job.

Finally, the study highlights that care workers who are not agency-based are the oldest subgroup of domestic workers, with a median age of 51. Since older people have a greater risk of severe illness from COVID-19, ultimately these workers are putting their own lives on the line to care for others.

Lack of regulations and invisibility

In addition to caring for children and helping households stay clean, domestic workers support the elderly, and people with disabilities or illnesses, by providing hands-on care, running errands, making meals, and cleaning homes. In this sense, domestic workers are incredibly valuable and make it possible for their employers to go to work and/or attend other obligations.

Despite domestic work being essential to our social reproductive life, the aforementioned data illustrate the devalued status of this type of industry that constantly faces low pay, rarely receives benefits, and has less access to full-time work than other workers. Because they work behind closed doors, particularly in private homes, they are away from public view and isolated from other workers, leaving them particularly susceptible to exploitation, mistreatment, and abuse from their employers. In addition, as mentioned in the introduction to this chapter, the majority of domestic workers are explicitly excluded from key federal labor laws and employment protections – a policy dating back to 1938, when majority Black domestic and farmworkers were excluded from landmark federal labor laws due to pressures from racist southern land-owners and lawmakers.

More specifically, domestic workers are excluded from the National Labor Relations Act (NLRA), enacted in 1935 to guarantee employees the right to form labor unions and organize for better working conditions; the Occupational Safety and Health Act (OSHA) does not apply to 'individuals who, in their own residences, privately employ persons for the purpose of performing … what are commonly regarded as ordinary domestic household tasks, such as house cleaning, cooking, and caring for children' and four federal anti-discrimination laws, such as the Civil Rights Act, the Americans with Disabilities Act, and the Age Discrimination in Employment Act. All of them generally cover only employers with multiple employees, thus, excluding the majority of domestic workers who work solo. This exclusion is also part of the Family and Medical Leave Act. Finally, 'live-in' workers are exempted from the overtime protections in the Fair Labor Standards Act, enacted in 1938.

Organizing and advocating efforts

In the US, it was not until 2010 that domestic workers slowly began to gain more recognition and rights as a work force. The first Bill of Rights for Domestic Workers was passed in New York, followed by California, Hawaii, Connecticut, Oregon, Nevada, Massachusetts, Illinois, New Mexico, the city of Seattle, and Virginia in early 2021. This bill ensures that domestic workers receive minimum wage, protections against sexual harassment, and the right to one day off if they work for more than 20 hours for an employer. However, it is taking a lot of time for this new legislation to be enforced and for domestic work to be recognized as any other type of work and be respected.

A critical first step to providing domestic workers with the same protections as other workers is passing a National

Domestic Workers Bill of Rights. In addition to extending basic wage and hour protections to domestic workers, establishing fair scheduling, transparent and comprehensive employment contracts, and access to health care and retirement benefits for domestic workers would be a significant improvement to their current working conditions.

NDWA, Hand in Hand, NY Caring Majority and affiliated groups, are organizations that have been working together and separately advocating for the rights and better working conditions of domestic workers in the United States. In addition, they organize to achieve the dignity, respect, and professionalism this work deserves. Yet, because of the COVID-19 pandemic, they all have sprung into immediate action. Over the course of the pandemic, tens of thousands of their NDWA members called representatives and senators demanding relief from the government. They have attended online and in-person actions and activities, supported and advocated for each other during these challenging times, and have built a community in spite of being physically distant (NDWA, 2020b). In particular, in response to the HEROES Act passed by the House of Representatives on May 15, 2020, the NDWA issued the following press release: 'The HEROES ACT includes significant provisions to bring domestic workers much of the relief they have been waiting for from the federal government, including billions of dollars in necessary relief to states and localities (…)' (NDWA, 2020c). Specifically, the HEROES Act, establishes key priorities for domestic workers including premium pay for a broad group of essential workers, financial assistance that is inclusive of millions of immigrant families, and expanded access to COVID-19 testing and treatment regardless of insurance coverage and citizenship status. These are critical and necessary steps towards improving working conditions and dignifying this work industry, especially in this time of crisis. In addition, in early 2021, NDWA, Hand in Hand, Adhikaar and Carroll Gardens Association petitioned New York City elected officials to adopt a new NYC Care Campaign platform that 'aims to transform NYC's care economy to one that is equitable and sustainable for all' (NDWA, 2021).

Employers

In terms of the employers' side of this social relationship, scholars, activists, and practitioners who are involved in the industry of care work, would largely agree that the relationship between employers and employees is complex due to the nature of this type of work (Sternberg, 2019). Across the Global North and South, domestic workers usually perform their work in a non-traditional workplace and behind closed doors, their work is widely unregulated, and has been historically devalued.

In addition, despite the fact that 'domestic work is work' explicitly stated in the 2011 International Labour Organization (ILO) convention no. 189, in many cases employers neither formally recognize domestic workers as legitimate 'workers', nor do they recognize themselves as employers (Hondagneu-Sotelo, 1997). There is a general perception among employers that their employees have special constitutional protections in a household setting compared to more traditional workplace settings where federal and state regulations do not fully apply (Young, 2010). Ultimately, the legal and professional relationship between employer and employee becomes blurred because neither party recognizes the household as the worker's formal work environment.

The complex relationship between employer and employee, aggravated during this pandemic, can be illustrated with the following example. In late 2020, Hand in Hand and NDWA New York hosted a conversation between employers and nannies to hear their experiences. During this conversation it was highlighted that those who are still employed are reporting ongoing difficulties negotiating PPE and necessary modifications to their work routine due to COVID-19. In addition, many nannies are being asked to take on additional responsibilities without being offered additional pay. This, of course, puts nannies in a very stressful situation as they are parents themselves who are struggling to balance work with caring for their own children. In other cases, nannies are reporting that employers are making demands that go beyond their work responsibilities. For example, it was reported that some employers in New York are requesting nannies to not use public transportation on their days off as a condition of employment (NDWA, 2020b).

Conclusion

First, it is imperative that employers increase the ability of domestic workers to practice social distancing without losing income and provide adequate PPE to domestic workers who are still cleaning, caring for children, and providing home care services in homes across the country. Here are three additional recommendations: employers should not expect or ask live-in domestic workers to perform tasks or jobs outside their regular tasks. For example, if a domestic worker was hired to take care of an elderly member in the home, that does not mean they are available to cook and clean. Employers should also create a simple, written contract that documents these terms as well as hours, work expectations, and tasks, and the employee should agree with these terms and sign the contract. Finally, employers should consider continuing to pay domestic workers during the pandemic even if they are unable to use their services due to social distancing.

Second, Congress must immediately pass the HEROES Act relief bill to begin to meet the urgent needs of working families. If passed, this legislation will send a strong signal that this workforce is essential for our social reproductive life and can no longer be overlooked. In the meantime, NDWA and organized domestic workers will continue to advocate to keep people connected to employment, to extend health care to all, to call for additional relief, and to create a real safety net and good jobs for everyone.

Finally, collective action matters, now more than ever.

References

Burnham, L. and Theodore, N. (2012) *Home Economics: The Invisible and Unregulated World of Domestic Work.* New York, NY: National Domestic Workers Alliance.

Hondagneu-Sotelo, P. (1997) 'Affluent players in the informal economy: employers of paid domestic workers'. *International Journal of Sociology and Social Policy*, 17(3/4): 130–58. https://doi.org/10.1108/eb013303

Lawson, V. (2007) 'Geographies of care and responsibility'. *Annals of the Association of American Geographers*, 97(1): 1–11.

National Domestic Workers Alliance (NDWA) (2020a) *Coronavirus' economic impact on domestic workers.* Retrieved from: https://domesticworkers.org/sites/default/files/Coronavirus_Report_4_8_20.pdf

National Domestic Workers Alliance (NDWA) (2020b) Press Releases. Retrieved from: www.domesticworkers.org

National Domestic Workers Alliance (NDWA) (2020c) Press Releases. Retrieved from: www.domesticworkers.org

National Domestic Workers Alliance (NDWA) (2021) Press Releases. Retrieved from: www.domesticworkers.org/release/coalition-domestic-worker-and-employer-groups-call-investment-paid-care-work

Sternberg, C. (2019) 'The hidden hand of domestic labor: domestic employers' work practices in Chicago, USA'. *Frontiers of Sociology*, 4: 6–11. DOI: 10.3389/fsoc.2019.00080

Wolfe, J., Kandra, J., Engdahl, L. and Shierholz, H. (2020) *Domestic Workers Chartbook: A Comprehensive Look at the Demographics, Wages, Benefits, and Poverty Rates of the Professionals who Care for our Family Members and Clean our Homes.* Washington, DC: Economy Policy Institute.

Young, D.E. (2010) 'The constitutional parameters of New York State's domestic workers bill of rights: balancing the rights of workers and employers'. *Albany Law Review*, 74: 1769–87.

50

Reflections of Living 'Hand-to-Mouth' among 'Hustlers' During COVID-19: Insights on the Realities of Poverty in Jamaica

Sheere Brooks

Introduction

This chapter considers effects of the first wave of the pandemic on 'hustling' activities due to government lock-down measures in Jamaica. Munive (2010) defines hustling as the everyday survival strategies of the marginalized to capitalize on opportunities to earn an income in extreme economic landscapes. In the spatial context of urban towns, hustling allows individuals to move around the city and make work, while building social ties (Thieme et al, 2021). Hustling is described as a risk–aversion strategy in the context of an unpredictable formal labor market, where diversification of income streams and economic opportunism is required for survival. Hustling is a livelihood mainly engaged in by poor and uneducated populations (Thieme, 2017). The informal labor market is defined as individuals who engage in productive activities that are not taxed or registered by the government.

Participants in the sector include self-employed laborers such as street vendors and sellers, own account workers, and labor hired informally. This particular definition takes into account the nature of hustling activities and conforms to a practice that generally occurs in developing countries (Charmes, 1990; see also Turner and Binh, Chapter Two; Thai et al, Volume 3). This is applicable to the Jamaican context.

The formal labor market in the Global South is unable to generate adequate employment opportunities, making hustling an important component of the informal labor market. The ILO (2020) highlighted the impacts of COVID-19 on informal workers in urban areas due to government lockdown measures.

The first section of this chapter will focus on the informal labor market in relation to the 'right to the city' in the urban Global South. A description of the methodological approach of the study will be followed by empirical evidence on the effects of the pandemic on hustling; the coping strategies of hustlers, and corresponding impacts on local businesses. Finally, the paper questions traditional approaches to assessing poverty and proposes an alternative approach that captures a realistic insight surrounding the precarity of hustling and risks to poverty.

Right to the city and hustling

'Urban governance' and 'right to the city' are concepts associated with the management of public space. Harvey (2008) defines the 'right to the city' in terms of the individual liberty to access urban space. Government authorities manage public spaces in ways designed to exclude certain groups; notably, homeless people, drug addicts, and loitering youth, in the Global North (see Turman et al, Volume 2; De Backer and Melgaço, Volume 3), and informal workers, in the Global South (Bal et al, Chapter Thirteen). Lindell (2008) observes that governments are expected to formalize the informal sector, eradicate poverty, and manage the urban economy, but this is steeped in western perceptions of what cities should look like, while criminalizing informal workers who use public spaces. In exploring the intersection between public space and informal livelihoods such as hustling, Nnkya (2004) and Brown (2006) attribute this tension to the design, governance, and management of cities. The spatial location of informal activities is essential to the minimization of distance, and purchasing of supplies and services, as well as spatial concentration. This allows a quick response to changes in consumer demand and tastes.

Background to the informal labor market in Jamaica

Jamaica is a Caribbean island (4,411 square miles), with a population of 2.8 million. The informal sector, excluding illegal activities, constitutes 43 percent of GDP (IDB, 2006). Explanations regarding the growth and pervasiveness of informal economic activity can be attributed to the continued decline of formal employment in the agriculture and bauxite/alumina sectors since the 1960s. The global crisis in 2008 led to a stagnation in earnings from tourism and reduced inflows of remittances, resulting in high unemployment in the country. Persistent slow growth of the Jamaican economy has reduced the availability of formal job opportunities, which is further compounded by low educational levels. Conversely, this has increased growth of the informal labor market (Statistical Institute of Jamaica, 2009).

'Hustling' as an informal livelihood in the Jamaican urban space

Hustling is a common livelihood strategy in Jamaica. In Jamaican parlance, the term, 'doing a business' implies many Jamaicans are trying to earn money through hustling (Davis, 2020). Hustling is a mobile activity and involves being in the most lucrative location for making a living. Hustling activities are itinerant and unregulated, mainly taking place though 'chance', while engaging in multiple sources of income in urban space by moving around. Unlike hustling, a street vendor is generally situated in a fixed location, but can experience the ire of local government officials and the police who can either seize goods or administer hefty fines. The street vendor may be an irritant to store owners, who feel inconvenienced by their encroachment and competition of stalls outside their stores, but a reciprocal arrangement can exist, whereby the street vendor sells 'hard to sell' goods on behalf of the store owner, while the latter offers 'protection' and authorizes the street vendor.

In Jamaica, participation in hustling activities is assessed in the country's labor force survey using proxy indicators. The survey defines the 'informal sector' in respect to non-agricultural activities, but the term 'hustling' is not used. A hustler who cultivates vegetables and sells them on the street may be construed as a non-agricultural worker, which is contradictory. The Economic and Social Survey of Jamaica (ESSJ) (Planning Institute of Jamaica, 2018) explained the extent of hustling by stating the number of people outside the labor force increased by 2.9 percent in 2018, when compared to 2017. The survey noted that there were 750,525 persons outside the labor force in 2018, of which 54.9 percent of respondents stated that 'they did not want to work'.[1] Other observations from the data shows that relative to males, 63.9 percent more females 'did not want to work'; 51.7 percent were 'incapable of work'; while 95.6 percent 'stayed home with dependents'. However, the general impression is that people may not want to engage in the formal labor market (perhaps through choice) and may find hustling to be convenient and flexible. The imprecise nature of measurement variables in the survey leaves responses open to 'speculation'. Many countries lack standardized data on informal labor and collect data through sector-specific surveys that do not accurately reflect household labor force participation (Banks,

2016). The fact that hustling is a popular livelihood strategy, compounded by a weak formal labor market, suggests that a sizable proportion of the population could be engaged in this activity, but the precise reasons cannot be determined.

Case study and research methodology

Annotto Bay is a principal urban town in the parish of St Mary, with a population of 114,227. Similar to the history of other Jamaican parishes, St Mary was formerly dominated by the plantation economy of sugar cane and banana production. During and after colonialism, Annotto Bay was an established and busy port town with a railway network and wharves that supported the agriculture industry. By the end of the twentieth century, the agrarian economy of the parish began to dissipate, compounded by the dismantling of agriculture preferential trade agreements with the European Union, the destruction of crops due to diseases, and the withdrawal of multinationals. This increased unemployment has made hustling and the informal labor market crucial to the survival of the population in Annotto Bay.

During the first wave of the pandemic, a lockdown of Annotto Bay began on May 7, 2020, and access into the town was restricted (Davis, 2020). The author was kept informed on the lockdown through informal discussions on the telephone with residents of the town, as well as reviewing the local media. Once lockdown was lifted on May 21, 2020, the author visited the town and safely held informal discussions with available hustlers and shop owners regarding impacts on livelihoods. Data collection methods also included observation and the use of secondary data sources. This methodological approach provided verification regarding the effects of the pandemic on hustlers and shop owners during the first wave of the pandemic when it was not ethically safe to conduct field research.

The impact of the pandemic and lock-down on 'hustling activities' in Annotto Bay

During the pandemic, a spike in the number of infections occurred in the town of Annotto Bay, which led to a lockdown of the town. The police and military prohibited access to the town, and commercial businesses were closed. The town is a thriving hub, providing transportation to other parts of the island. Hustlers are dependent on commercial businesses for goods to re-sell to the public. Hustling in the town is most lucrative when shoppers and travelers are in the town. In the absence of customers, hustlers could not purchase goods for resale. During the lockdown, hustlers complained of being 'hungry' with no source of livelihood to be generated.

Grocery stores described experiencing reduced sales due to the loss of custom from hustlers unable to purchase food items from the stores. Hustling in an urban town can involve being on the streets for long periods at a time. Whatever income is earned during the morning can be used to purchase a breakfast meal, usually consisting of slices of bread (referred to as 'half or a quarter loaf of bread'; two eggs, and a tea bag to make a cup of tea). By lunchtime, the hustler patronizes the same shop to purchase lunch items (for example tinned meat or fish, cheese or bread or crackers, and a beverage). By the evening, hustlers would again patronize the same store to purchase items for a dinner meal (for example fresh meat or tinned meat/fish, rice or flour, and a beverage).[2] Restrictions on entering urban towns was detrimental to hustling activities. A report on the impact of COVID-19 on livelihoods in Jamaica showed there was widespread disruption to livelihoods primarily owing to movement restrictions and transport limitations[3] (United Nations World Food Programme (UNWFP), 2020). Another observation was the existence of a reciprocal arrangement between the grocery store owners and the hustler, as the former is dependent on the latter to patronize the store while retaining a regular customer base from among the hustlers.

Conclusion

Hustling is a survival strategy that commonly occurs in urban towns in the Global South. The impact of the pandemic in Jamaica revealed the hardships experienced. This raises questions regarding the capacity of existing poverty measures to include periods of shock (such as the pandemic) as livelihoods are constrained. The Jamaica Survey of Living Conditions (JSLC) is an annual household survey that focuses on poverty and consumption. On a rotating basis, the survey focuses on coping strategies, but this not a regular assessment. Existing poverty assessment is narrowly based on an absolute measure, using the cost of food and non-food items in a basket to calculate the poverty line. The poverty line determines whether a person is below the poverty line to determine risk to poverty (Statistical Institute of Jamaica, 2009, 2014, 2018). In the context of this study, a hustler may be able to afford items in the food basket and are therefore not deemed as poor, but the JSLC does not take into account vulnerabilities surrounding hustling activities, such as those periods when livelihoods are curtailed due to spatial closures and lockdowns in urban towns.

The pandemic revealed the coping strategies of the poor. This raises the need for a complementary poverty measurement that regularly maps out the coping strategies used by the poor to survive. It is likely that the next round of the JSLC survey will not take place until 2022, and so documentation of the experience of poverty and coping strategies during the pandemic may not occur based on the passage of time. The popularity of hustling as a livelihood strategy in Jamaica warrants a re-think about existing statistical approaches to assessing the number of people in poverty and a joined-up approach in collecting data that documents the lived experience of hustlers and their survival. This will be important for documenting lesson-learning experiences and transfer to poverty alleviation policies.

The buildup of social capital between hustlers and formal businesses is a survival tactic, as evidenced by a symbiotic and dependent relationship, essential to establishing interconnections to safeguard livelihoods. One possible poverty alleviation approach is to change existing negativities about the informal sector by implementing measures to transform hustling into a legitimate business and entrepreneurial concern in the Global South. The idea that there exists a gap between formal and informal entities may be unfounded, as the challenges of the pandemic revealed that both entities are dependent on each other for survival.

Notes

[1] ESSJ analysis generally shows that the majority of people outside of the labor force are females, aged 25–54 years.

[2] The cost of these items would be far less than buying cooked food (referred to as 'box food' in Jamaican parlance) from a cook shop. The absence of fresh fruit and vegetables from these meals may not necessarily be an indication of nutritional deficiency, as a hustler may obtain unsold fruits and vegetables from a vendor's stall.

[3] The data from this report was restricted to just 'livelihoods' and was not disaggregated to informal livelihoods. Secondly, the report provided an overview of impacts arising from COVID-19, but the data was not representative, as the use of a web-based questionnaire limited inputs from respondents without internet connectivity.

References

Banks, N. (2016) 'Youth poverty, employment and livelihoods: social and economic implications of living with insecurity in Arusha, Tanzania'. *Environment and Urbanisation*, 28(2): 437–54.

Brown, A. (2006) *Contested Space: Street Trading, Public Space and Livelihoods in Developing Cities*. Warwickshire: ITDG Publishing.

Charmes, J. (1990) 'A critical review of concepts, definitions and research on the informal sector', in D. Turnham, B. Salom and A. Schwartz (eds) *The Informal Sector Revisited*. Paris: OECD Development Centre Seminars, pp 11–51.

Davis, G. (2020) 'Normality returns to Annotto Bay as St Mary quarantine expires'. *The Jamaica Gleaner*, May 23.

Harvey, D. (2008) 'The right to the city'. *New Left Review*, 53: 23–40.

Inter-American Development Bank (IDB) (2006) *The informal sector in Jamaica*. Washington DC: Inter-American Development Bank.

International Labour Organization (ILO) (2014) *Informal employment in Jamaica: notes on formalization ILO Regional Office for Latin America and the Caribbean*. Retrieved from: www.ilo.org/wcmsp5/groups/public/---americas/---ro-lima/documents/publication/wcms_245888.pdf

International Labour Organization (ILO) (2020) *ILO Monitor: COVID-19 and the world of work*. Updated estimates and analysis. 2nd edition. Retrieved from: www.ilo.org/global/topics/coronavirus/impacts-and-responses/WCMS_767028/lang--en/index.htm

Lindell, I. (2008) 'The multiple sites of urban governance: insights from an African City'. *Urban Studies*, 45(9): 1879–901.

Munive, J. (2010) 'The army of "unemployed" young people'. *Young – Nordic Journal of Youth Research*, 18(3): 321–38.

Nnkya, T. (2004) *A rights-based approach: governance, context & experience of public space and livelihoods in Dar es Salaam: preliminary research report*. Cardiff: Cardiff School of City and Regional Planning.

Planning Institute of Jamaica (2018) *Economic and social survey of Jamaica*. Kingston: Planning Institute of Jamaica.

Statistical Institute of Jamaica (2009) *Jamaica survey of living conditions*. Kingston: Statistical Institute of Jamaica.

Statistical Institute of Jamaica (2014) *Jamaica survey of living conditions*. Kingston: Statistical Institute of Jamaica.

Statistical Institute of Jamaica (2018) *Jamaica survey of living conditions*. Kingston: Statistical Institute of Jamaica.

Thieme, T. (2017) 'The hustle economy: informality, uncertainty and the geographies of getting by'. *Progress in Human Geography*, 42(4): 1–20.

Thieme, T., Ference, M. and van Stapele, N. (2021) '"Harnessing the Hustle": struggle, solidarities and narratives of work in Nairobi and beyond'. *Africa*, 91 (1): 1–15.

United Nations World Food Programme (UNWFP) (2020) *Caribbean COVID-19 food security and livelihoods impact survey: Jamaica summary report, May 2020*. Christ Church, Barbados.

SIX

Looking at Urban Inequalities Regarding Different Jobs in the Age of COVID-19: Who Stayed at Home, Who Did Not?

Ferhan Gezici and Cansu İlhan

Introduction

The diverging trajectories in economic activities stemming from pandemic prevention measures (such as working from home directives) continues to affect sectors and employees worldwide in different ways (see Shearmur et al, Volume 4). According to data from the June 2020 Global Economic Prospects Report, in the best-case scenario, the COVID-19 pandemic pushed 71 million people below the poverty line, drawing the extreme poverty rate to 8.82 percent (World Bank, 2020). Although lockdowns impacted almost all sectors, those impacts varied across employment and economic sectors. A study conducted in the United States revealed that some sectors, such as trade, passenger transport, arts and entertainment, accommodation, food and beverage, and other personal services, were comparatively more affected. Some occupational groups working in different positions within these sectors were also affected in different ways. Employees in these sectors are younger and less well-educated, with lower annual income, thus making them economically less secure during the COVID-19 pandemic (Berube and Bateman, 2020).

The pandemic has deepened inequalities, both in terms of the economic loss (dependent to some extent on the ability or inability to work from home) and the disease risk to those who continue to go to work. Frontline workers in health care and critical supply chains continue to work under the risk of infection, although they are less financially affected (Bergamini, 2020). While economic activities have slowed down worldwide, the capacity to work remotely determines the extent of the economic costs caused by the pandemic. The ability to work remotely depends on the nature of the jobs and employees. For example, academics may continue working in distance education, whereas employees at the same universities who provide catering services, stationery supplies, and so on may be adversely affected (OECD, 2020). According to statistics put forward in the United States, there is a strong relationship between income percentiles and rates of working from home. While the employees at the bottom of the income percentiles (bottom 25 percent) can work from home at a rate of 9.2 percent, this rate rises to 61.5 percent in the top quintile (top 25 percent) (Bergamini, 2020).

According to the OECD report, which evaluated the capabilities of remote work, the capacity to work from home in Turkey is around 21 percent, while it is 30 percent in Istanbul, the country's largest city (OECD, 2020). Working from home provides an opportunity to reduce the costs caused by the pandemic; however, not all professions are suitable for working from home (Özgüzel et al, 2020). Aytun and Özgüzel (2020) revealed that 24 percent of jobs in the private sector in Turkey are suitable for working remotely, which corresponds to 31 percent of the total wages. In addition to this, 70 percent of managers and professional occupational groups can work from home, while the corresponding rate is below 10 percent for occupations that do not require education qualifications.

The sectoral differentiation between the provinces in Turkey, the heterogeneity of labor quality, and the fact that large cities house professions that are more suitable to home-based work in greater numbers than rural areas (OECD, 2020) suggest that such an analysis will yield more meaningful results at the provincial level. Thus, this study is focused on Istanbul, which is the economic engine of the country, generating one third of the national GDP and housing one fifth of the total population. This study looks at changes in working conditions due to the pandemic, focusing on sectoral, spatial, and occupational groups. It based on the results of a survey conducted between April 15 and May 4, 2020, in Istanbul, soon after the pandemic broke out in Turkey. For the purposes of this study, 375 questionnaires were collected through social media in 36 districts of Istanbul. The results of the study reveal findings regarding the distribution of sectors and occupational groups who can and cannot work from home in districts, and the spatial concentration of occupational groups. The distribution of the questionnaires was made randomly and was not based on any pre-selection. The fact that the study was conducted in a short time period reveals a limited view on the long-term impacts of the pandemic on employment practices. However, it provides us with a clear picture of the first wave of the pandemic, and how it impacted working conditions across different sectors and different parts of the city.

Who stayed at home, who did not?

While 9.2 percent of the respondents in the survey conducted for the study are employers, 90.8 percent are paid employees. During the pandemic, 19.5 percent of the respondents continued working full-time on site, 16 percent worked on site part-time or by turns, 38.8 percent worked from home,

6.2 percent were on paid leave, 4.6 percent lost their jobs, 10.5 percent were forced to take unpaid leave, and 4.3 percent were business owners who closed their business. The highest number of those on unpaid leave and businesses shut down was observed in the arts, entertainment and recreation, wholesale and retail trade, and accommodation and food services sectors. Five sectors that stand out in the survey are manufacturing, wholesale and retail, finance and insurance, education, and health care. When analyzing the rate of working from home in these five prominent sectors, respondents in finance and insurance (68.8 percent) and education (65 percent) were more likely to work from home. Given their critical role during the pandemic, employees in health care went to work on site at a rate of 84.8 percent, while the rate of going to work in manufacturing (55.5 percent) and trade (34 percent) were moderate, causing significant differences between occupational groups.

We found that 90 percent of those who were working from home were managers, professional, and assistant professional group members. Considering the distribution of occupational groups of those who continued to work on site during the pandemic, the rate of managers and professionals was 50 percent, and the rate of employees in service and sales personnel and elementary occupations increased.

In the manufacturing sector, where the rate of going to work was high, employees, technicians, and operators in elementary occupations continued to work on site, while professional occupational groups in this sector were able to stay at home. As a result, as the rates of working from home and going to work can vary depending on the sector, the main determinant has been the positions of the employees within the sector.

During the pandemic, employees in education could mostly work from home at a rate of 65 percent, whereas 15 percent were on paid leave, and 7.5 percent were on unpaid leave or were dismissed. Professional groups made up 97.5 percent of the employees in education, while 2.5 percent were managers.

The rate of going to work in the health care sector, which has been the most crucial during the pandemic, was 84.9 percent. Only 0.9 percent of those have the opportunity to work from home in health care, and they are not health care personnel but engineers and managers employed in health care institutions.

Spatial differentiation

When our survey was analyzed by districts within Istanbul, five districts stand out as having the highest percentage of people able to work from home: Sarıyer, Ataşehir, Kadıköy, Beşiktaş, and Şişli. Three of these (Şişli, Beşiktaş, and Kadıköy) are the most developed districts of Istanbul in terms of socio-economic development, while Sarıyer and Ataşehir are ranked 11th and 13th respectively, out of the citys' 39 districts.

The rate of working from home varies according to their occupational composition. In Kadıköy, the percentage of professional occupations and managers is 65,8 percent. These are similarly high in the other districts with the highest percentage of those working from home: 80 percent in Beşiktaş; 64,3 percent in Şişli; 87,5 percent in Ataşehir; and 71,4 percent in Sarıyer. Districts with higher numbers of professionals and managers due to their education and skills could stay at home at higher rates. It should be noted that the districts with the greatest percentage of the workforce working from home can be found close to the Central Business Area, where many White-collar, professional jobs can be found (see Figure 6.1). On the other hand, the concentration of production and industrial areas can be found on the periphery, where we also observe the lowest rates of working from home. Again, as the socio-economic development index (SEDI) level decreases, it is observed that the rate of working from home decreases and the rate of going to work increases (Figure 6.1). In the meantime, we should consider the income heterogeneity within the same district in order to capture the pattern of inequalities.

Figure 6.1: Socio-economic development level of districts in Istanbul and percentage staying home

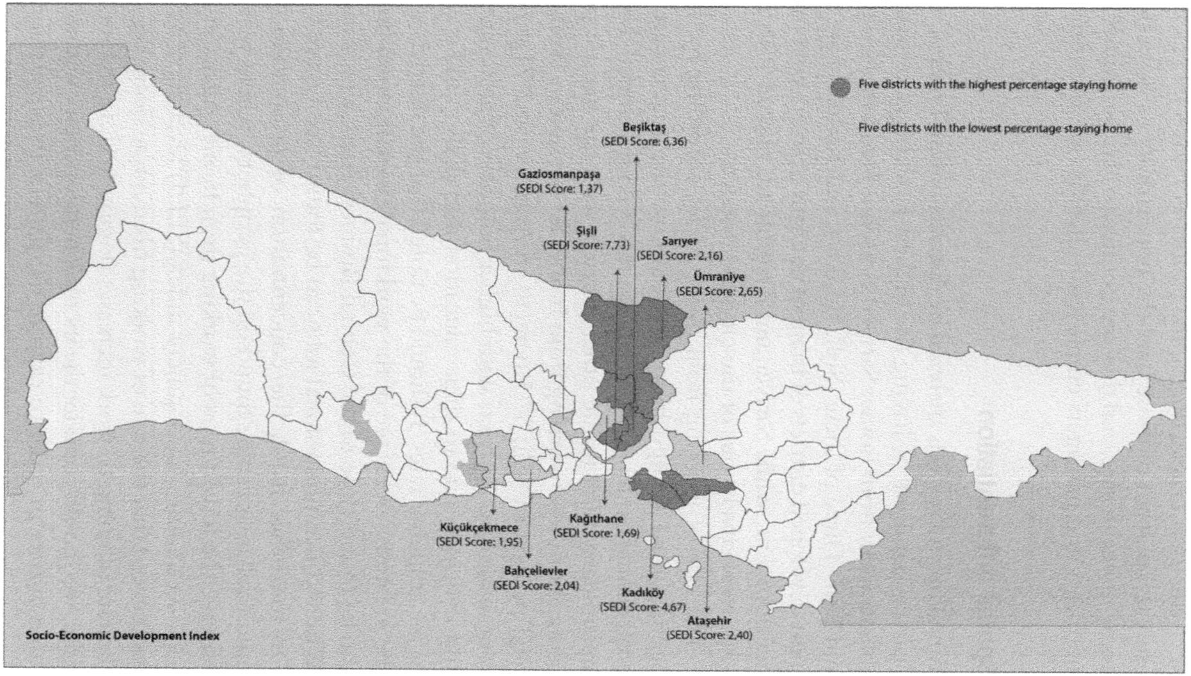

Source: Ministry of Industry and Technology (2019)

Conclusion

The easing of the first lockdown began gradually in Turkey, on May 11, 2020. Thus, the results presented in this study summarize the outlook before normalization. Istanbul, with its large population and strong economy, became the center of the pandemic in Turkey, in line with other global cities during the initial phase of the pandemic. Working from home was considered an opportunity for a densely populated metropolitan city in order to reduce mobility and the risk of disease. Our findings show spatial and sectoral inequalities that have amplified the pre-existing inequalities within Istanbul. This is not only about jobs and the ability to work from home, but also in terms of the risk of being exposed to COVID-19 through performing work on site and other factors such as the need to take crowded public transport to get to work each day. On the one hand, well-educated, skilled, and high wage employees are more likely to be able to work remotely. In addition to this, they also have the opportunity to advance their careers. On the other hand, not only the nature of jobs, but the suitability of space and technological infrastructure of residents to work from home, have furthered inequalities (such as having reliable home internet). Furthermore, considering cultural factors, gender inequalities have gradually become a significant consequence of the pandemic, since women are more likely to be responsible for childcare while working from home (for more on gender-based inequalities, see Chapters 13 and 20).

Trends and patterns both before and during the pandemic indicate that digital transformations that enable some people to work from home will continue to accelerate as we move into the post-pandemic period. This can further widen the existing socio-economic inequalities due to varying rates of access to technical infrastructure facilities. In particular, education has been one of the areas where access to the internet and capacity has become the most controversial. With the start of distance education, the uneven nature of household access to the necessary technological equipment and the internet has further exacerbated inequalities in education, along many of the same lines as employment. It is estimated that 1.5 million students do not have internet access and therefore have little ability to access distance education in Turkey. On the other hand, the number of students taking private lessons (via the internet and video conferencing) has increased (Eğitim-Sen, 2020).

As a result, the pandemic has led to variegated effects both in terms of different sectors and for employees in different positions within each sector. When it comes to the question on how people survive, it is apparent that those who have the opportunity to work from home will remain resilient as long as they received their salaries. However, the intensification of the economic crisis and inflation remain major concerns. Those who lost all or part of their income (part-time employees and those on unpaid leave) have tried to survive by relying on their pre-pandemic savings and taking on debts during the pandemic. As a final comment, Istanbul is somewhat of an outlier within Turkey, since it has the country's greatest proportion of people working remotely. However, growing economic and employment inequalities are evident throughout the country and must therefore be a major focus for policy makers now and in the post-pandemic period.

Note

The authors would like to thank the students of the Urban Economics course (2019–2020 spring term) at the Urban and Regional Planning Department at ITU who conducted the surveys.

References

Aytun, U. and Özgüzel, C. (2020) 'Turkiye'nin evden calismasi mumkun mu?', April 12. https://sarkac.org/2020/04/turkiyenin-evden-calismasi-mumkun-mu/

Bergamini, E. (2020) 'How COVID-19 is laying bare inequality', March 31. www.bruegel.org/2020/03/how-covid-19-is-laying-bare-inequality/

Berube, A. and Bateman, N. (2020) 'Who are the workers already impacted by the COVID-19 recession?' April 3. www.brookings.edu/research/who-are-the-workers-already-impacted-by-the-covid-19-recession/

Eğitim-Sen (2020) *Salgın Günlerinde Uzaktan Eğitim Çalıştayı Sonuç Raporu*. Eğitim-Sen. https://egitimsen.org.tr/wp-content/uploads/2020/09/sonuç-raporu.pdf

OECD (2020) *Capacity for remote working can affect shutdowns' costs differently across places*, OECD COVID-19 Policy Note. www.oecd.org/coronavirus/policy-responses/capacity-for-remote-working-can-affect-lockdown-costs-differently-across-places-0e85740e/

Özgüzel, C., Veneri, P. and Ahrend, R. (2020) 'Potential for remote working across different places', July 15. https://voxeu.org/article/potential-remote-working-across-different-places

World Bank (2020) *Projected poverty impacts of COVID-19*. www.worldbank.org/en/topic/poverty/brief/projected-poverty-impacts-of-COVID-19

PART II

Life During Lockdown

Ageist Transport Infrastructures: Rethinking Public Transport amid COVID-19 Lockdowns in India

Prajwal Nagesh, Ajay Bailey, Sobin George, and

Lekha Subaiya

Introduction

The hypermobile cities of India stood still with the onset of COVID-19-induced lockdowns. Public transport services were the first to be suspended, and older adults in particular were instructed not to leave their homes (Press Information Bureau (PIB), 2020). Even with the easing of lockdown and the resumption of limited public transport, older adults were 'restricted' from using services as per the pandemic-related advisories issued by the state. Mobility, which is central to active aging, health status, and well-being (World Health Organization (WHO), 2007) of older adults, was affected by this exclusion in the public transport system. The short- and medium-term implications of such lockdown protocols towards the (im)mobility of older adults requires attention. Given the Indian urban transport scenario, the dependence of older adults (particularly those from low-income groups) on public transport and the inadequate public transport infrastructure is relevant to contextualize the pandemic advisories.

This chapter uses the case of Bengaluru city in southern India to highlight how transport protocols issued during the COVID-19 pandemic impacted older adults' (im)mobility. Even before the lockdown was rolled out on March 24, 2020, Bengaluru's public transport system had been struggling to cater to passenger demand. With physical distancing norms in place, which reduced ridership and trip number, it has become more difficult for passengers in general, and older adult passengers in particular, to access public transport. In Bengaluru, a large proportion of older adults are mobile, work in the informal sector, and earn a low income. They cannot afford private transportation and are therefore dependent on public transport (Baindur and Rao, 2016). The exclusion of this group from the public transport system will have implications for their access to work, social life, and essentials such as banking, health care, and groceries.

In this chapter, we take an intersectional perspective, where we examine how events such as the COVID-19 pandemic further accentuated the already disadvantageous position of older adults in the absence of age-friendly interventions. The chapter reviews the literature, government circulars, and social media communication to understand the state's major transport-related decisions. We use data from our online survey (conducted between June 9 and June 30, 2020), in which we focused on the impact of COVID-19 lockdowns on older adults' mobility in urban India. The 172 responses received from older adults living in Bengaluru city are the basis of the analysis in this chapter. The absence of a sampling framework due to the survey's online nature will remain a limitation of representativeness.

Transport policies and ageism during COVID-19

Public transport is at the core of the city's geography and is vital to the mobility of older adults. Bus and metro rail are the most common modes of transport within Bengaluru's public transit system. Even before the COVID-19 pandemic, Bengaluru's public transport system struggled to cater to four million passenger trips per day with an inadequate fleet of 6,162 buses run by the Bangalore Metropolitan Transport Corporation (BMTC) and a mere 42 km metro network administered by the Bangalore Metro Rail Corporation Limited (BMRCL). The abrupt lockdown on March 24, 2020 led to an immediate suspension of public transport services (see Figure 7.1). Since May 19, 2020, the BMTC has been operating with a fraction of its fleet, and the metro rail resumed with depleted services after a five-month break. The ad hoc transport decisions might have been well-intended, but are counterproductive as they are not in tune with the travel needs, the precarity of livelihoods, and the centrality of public transport to older adults' life activities.

Researchers worldwide have argued that the narrative of ageism has accompanied pandemic advisories in general (Fraser et al, 2020; Lindenberg et al, Chapter 19; Hartt et al, Volume Four). We further extend this argument for urban public transport. A critical analysis of Bengaluru's transport advisories (see Figure 7.1) during the pandemic highlights a few problematic elements. First, the series of transport measures were prohibitive rather than suggestive. The language of 'restriction' and 'instruction' serves into ageist narratives of older persons needing to be protected. The BMRCL, in its circular on March 20, 2020 (even before the lockdown), stated that persons above 60 years are 'restricted from travel' in the metro (Bangalore Metro Rail Corporation Limited (BMRCL), 2020). The BMTC, which resumed operations in phases, continued to prohibit the use of its service by persons above 65 years of age (*The Hindu*, 2020). The agency of older adults to make

Figure 7.1: Timeline of state response concerning public transport during the COVID-19 pandemic, March 24–September 30, 2020

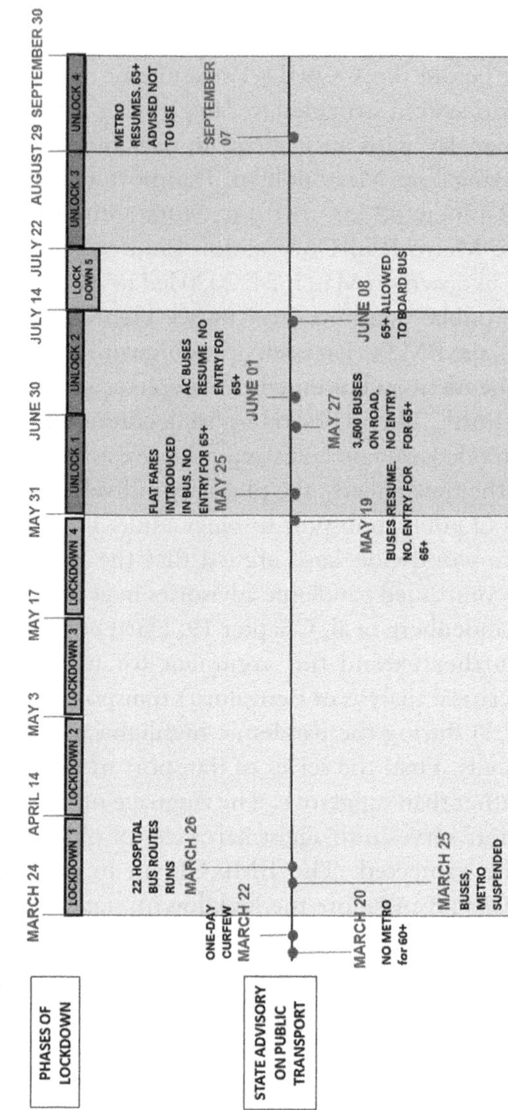

Note: The word Unlock is as used by BBMP (2020) in its circulars. Unlock refers to the phased lifting of COVID-19-related lockdown restrictions.

Source: Author's representation

decisions about their safety was forsaken, with their livelihoods put at risk by restricting their mobility. Second, the consideration of age as a single dimension category portrays older adults as a homogenous, vulnerable, and at-risk group. There are variations in the nature of employment, living arrangements, and health care needs of older persons, all of which generate different mobility needs. A blanket restriction ignoring the intersectional categories and needs of older adults is likely to disrupt the life activities of the most vulnerable among them. Chronological age used as the single criterion for risk classification leads to 'unfair and unacceptable' ageist policies (Rahman and Jahan, 2020). Third, there is a lack of consensus as to who is a senior citizen. Whether this constitutes persons above 60 years or 65 years is not clear from the contradicting advisories of BMTC and BMRCL (see Figure 7.1). Both the transit agencies, catering to the same population in a single city, lack coherence in defining the 'senior citizen'. This can lead to inconsistent information for older adults to access public transport. Older adults already suffering from inaccessible transport were further immobilized by these ambiguities.

Immobilizing the vulnerable

The World Health Organization guidelines for active ageing in an age-friendly city proposed that policies and systems respect older adults' decisions and lifestyle choices (WHO, 2007). Contrarily, the condescending attitude of transport policies during the pandemic produced psychosocial concerns and endangered their livelihoods. Our online survey among older adults in Bengaluru showed that, as a result of lockdown, there was a steep decrease in the use of public transport (Figure 7.2).

Webber et al (2010) argued that for older adults, activity reduction from a lack of mobility could lead to physical deconditioning, reduced social participation, and affects health and well-being. Similar concerns emerge from the restrictions on the mobility of older adults during the pandemic. The

Figure 7.2: Public transport usage and perceptions of safety by older adults during the pandemic

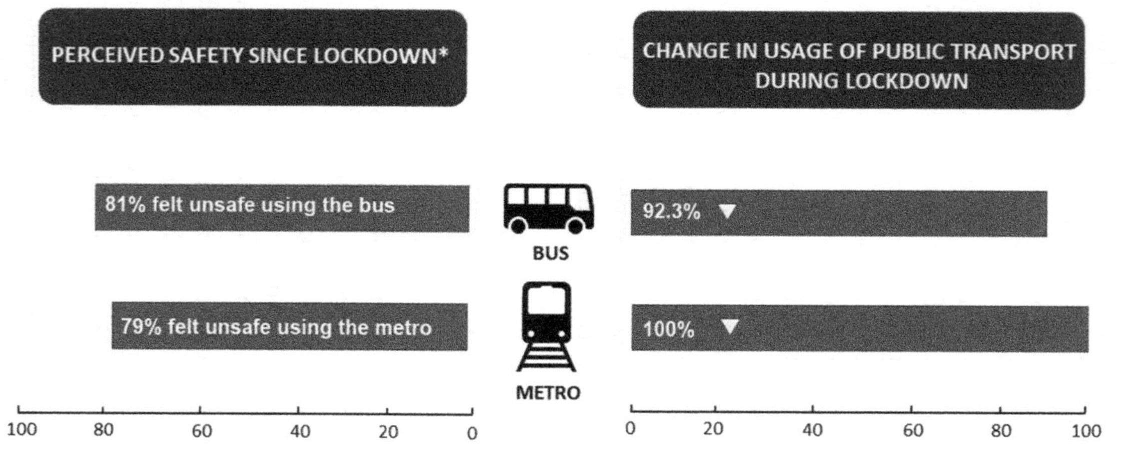

* **Lockdown refers to March 24, 2020 when the pan-India lockdown came into force**

Source: Author's representation using the data from the online survey

survey showed that the use of bus and metro rail service by older adults had plummeted to almost nil after the lockdown in March 2020 (Figure 7.2). Of serious concern is the heightened perception of public transport being unsafe. The belief that public transport is unsafe, particularly for older adults, is likely to curb their mobility. These regulations have meant that routine trips to work, grocery shops, parks, religious places are restricted. Consequently, connections beyond one's house – the neighborhood, the extended family, the community, and the society at large – were affected. Almost all the older adults who participated in the survey reported that they did not meet friends or neighbors during the lockdown. More than a third of older adults reported feeling down, depressed, and hopeless; 46 percent said they felt nervous or stressed, and 50 percent said they had little interest or pleasure in doing things during the lockdown. Immobility and lack of digital literacy can combine to make it difficult for older adults to maintain social relationships, which could produce other psychosocial concerns. Therefore, considering age as the solitary factor to identify risk groups will not only make them immobile but will further the long-standing problem of social isolation in cities (Armitage and Nellums, 2020; Fraser et al, 2020).

Recent literature (such as Bhan et al, 2020) has shown that lockdown protocols enforced during the pandemic have weak roots, given the realities of Indian cities. Unlike in western cities, many older adults in cities of the Global South such as Bengaluru live with scarce resources; they work in the informal sector well beyond formal retirement age and rely on a patchwork of public infrastructure and services. 'Work from home', 'order from home', and 'stay at home' protocols do not apply to many who work as daily wage laborers in markets, as security guards, as domestic maids, or in unorganized small-scale industries (Bhan et al, 2020; see also Lemanski and De Groot, Chapter Ten). Digital literacy among older adults is much lower than the population as a whole, and poorer older adults have limited access to such technology (Khokhar, 2016). Given this context, the sole reliance on technology to order essentials, work, and obtain information on policies shows an ageist attitude. From this perspective, stigmatization and restrictions in the use of public transport only worsen the ability of older persons to earn a decent livelihood. We argue that during the pandemic, the decisions made by governing bodies have been overarching and not contextual. The realities on the ground in developing countries, such as the lack of universal access to technology, health infrastructure, and care systems, have been ignored in lockdown policies. The top-down epidemiological responses to the pandemic of abrupt lockdowns and ad-hoc restrictions on older adults' mobility may have been meant to protect them but have only exacerbated the precarious nature of their living conditions (see also Lemanski and de Groot, Chapter Ten).

Conclusion

The prospect of improving transport access for older adults is already confronted with depleted services and insufficient funding. The decline in operations during the COVID-19 lockdown has reduced fare box revenue, the primary income source for transit agencies. The financial situation of these already debt-ridden public transport bodies is further affected. In this context, the state has been defensive about public transport policy and funding. Fares have been increased, the fleet has been reduced, and concessions for older adults have been withdrawn. The gradual progress made over time on equitable transport policies is under threat of being eroded.

Learning from these experiences, we make the following recommendations for future transport policies under such emergencies. First, we note that the consequences of the denial of transport infrastructures to older adults (determined solely based on age) are equally important as COVID-19 prevention since they will be exposed to the risks of social isolation, loss of livelihood, and lack of access to essential services. Second, the abrupt and stringent lockdown on transport services needs to be reviewed critically from the dimension of ageism. Transport policies should avoid ageist restrictions or the prohibition of older adults from accessing public transport. Instead, we propose that there is a need to provide safe, accessible, and prioritized travel options to older adults in place of protectionist policies. Mobility, particularly on public transport, is key for active ageing, and this needs to be the fundamental underpinning while undertaking policy decisions hereafter.

Note

This work is part of the research project 'Inclusive Cities through Equitable access to Urban Mobility Infrastructures for India and Bangladesh' (PI: A. Bailey) under the research program Joint Sustainable Development Goal research initiative with project number W 07.30318.003, which is financed by the Dutch Research Council (NWO) and Utrecht University, the Netherlands.

References

Armitage, R. and Nellums, L.B. (2020) 'COVID-19 and the consequences of isolating the elderly'. *The Lancet Public Health*, 5(5): e256.

Baindur, D. and Rao, P. (2016) 'Equity in public transport: a case of Bangalore's city bus transport'. *Journal of Sustainable Urbanization, Planning and Progress*, 1(1).

Bangalore Metro Rail Corporation Limited (BMRCL) (2020) Bangalore Metro advisory on COVID-19. Retrieved from: https://rb.gy/mihpif

BBMP (The Bruhat Bengaluru Mahanagara Palike) (2020) *BBMP COVID-19 Bulletin*. Retrieved from: https://dl.bbmpgov.in/covid/Covid_Bengaluru_12August_2020 Bulletin-142 English.pdf

Bhan, G., Caldeira, T., Gillespie, K. and Simone, A. (2020) 'The pandemic, southern urbanisms and collective life'. *Society and Space*. www.societyandspace.org/articles/the-pandemic-southern-urbanisms-and-collective-life

Fraser, S., Lagacé, M., Bongué, B. et al (2020) 'Ageism and COVID-19: what does our society's response say about us?' *Age and Ageing*, 49(5): 692–5.

Khokhar, A.S. (2016) 'Digital literacy: how prepared is India to embrace it?' *International Journal of Digital Literacy and Digital Competence*, 7(3).

Press Information Bureau (PIB) (2020) Retrieved from: https://pib.gov.in/PressReleseDetail.aspx?PRID=1607248

Rahman, A. and Jahan, Y. (2020) 'Defining a "risk group" and ageism in the era of COVID-19'. *Journal of Loss and Trauma*, 25(8): 631–4.

The Hindu (2020) 'Senior citizens can now travel in BMTC buses'. Retrieved from: https://rb.gy/ecwepw

Webber, S.C., Porter, M.M. and Menec, V.H. (2010) 'Mobility in older adults: a comprehensive framework'. *Gerontologist*, 50(4): 443–50.

World Health Organization (WHO) (2007) *Global age-friendly cities: a guide*. Geneva, Switzerland: WHO.

EIGHT

The Pandemic and Food Insecurity in Small Cities of the Global South: A Case Study of Noapara in Bangladesh

M. Feisal Rahman and Hanna A. Ruszczyk

Introduction

The unfolding economic and social consequences of the COVID-19 pandemic has exposed fault lines in existing food systems in both developed (Lawrence, 2020) and developing countries (Rahman et al, 2020). Bangladesh, a densely populated and rapidly urbanizing nation of roughly 180 million people went into a 'general holiday with restrictions on movement' (referred to internationally as lockdown) on March 26, 2020. The majority of economic and social activities within the country ceased as a consequence. The lockdown was eventually relaxed on June 1, 2020, with specific instructions to maintain social distancing. As of September 7, 2020, Bangladesh had 325,157 cases of COVID-19 and 4,479 people had died from the virus (Directorate General of Health Services (DGHS), 2020). A rapid-response research conducted by the Power and Participation Research Centre and BRAC

Institute of Governance and Development of Bangladesh (Rahman et al, 2020) in April 2020 in Bangladesh observed a steep drop in income leading to a contraction in food consumption as evidenced by reduction in food expenditure by 28 percent for urban informal settlement respondents and 22 percent for rural respondents. Similar to experiences in other countries (Despard et al, 2020), the lockdown resulted in an income shock, particularly for the urban poor.

While there are reports of how communities in major cities have been impacted (Taylor, 2020), little is known about the lived experiences of residents in smaller cities and how food systems and food security in these towns were impacted. Indeed, small and mid-sized cities remain academically and professionally ignored and unexplored despite the fact that the world's urban majority reside in those cities (Satterthwaite, 2017; Ruszczyk et al, 2021). The relationship between food security, food systems, and sustainability also needs engaged consideration within these small cities (Mackay, 2019). Understanding this relationship is crucial because urban poverty and food insecurity are inter-related. Tacoli (2019) explains that most urban residents not only need to purchase the majority of their food but, unlike in rural areas, it is their main expenditure. Local governments in small cities also have curtailed capacity, minimal funding under their control, and often lack political power to fulfill their responsibilities. These pre-existing socio-economic conditions indicate that food security and food systems in small cities were also likely impacted by the pandemic-induced lockdown.

In order to address this knowledge gap, a rapid assessment study focusing on two small cities, namely Mongla and Noapara, in southwestern Bangladesh was undertaken. This chapter will share findings from the data collected from Noapara before, during, and immediately after the lockdown. In doing so, the chapter will delineate the challenges imposed by COVID-19 on food (in)security in Noapara and also identify associated coping mechanisms undertaken by affected residents.

Methodology

The study was conducted in collaboration with the International Centre for Climate Change and Development (ICCCAD) based in Dhaka, Bangladesh. The study team conducted a rapid assessment to understand how low- and middle-income residents in small cities such as Noapara were coping. Between May and July 2020, the team conducted 15 formal, telephone-based, semi-structured interviews undertaken with selected key informants from Noapara to understand their lived experiences of the lockdown and the effect the lockdown had on the food security of residents in the city (Rahman and Ruszczyk, 2020; Ruszczyk et al, 2020). The study also builds on research (ICCCAD, 2020a) on life in small cities which is based on 200 surveys, 40 interviews and storytelling workshops conducted between September 2019 and March 2020. These key informants of the present study represent a cross-section of residents (from low-income households and from middle-class families, men and women), stakeholders, and government officials with whom we engaged during the autumn 2019 fieldwork.

Pre-pandemic food and nutritional environment in Noapara

Noapara is a thriving city, serving an important national transportation function. It has a national transportation road bisecting the city, and the railway links Noapara to the rest of Bangladesh as well as to India. The Bhairav River at Noapara connects Noapara as a river port to the seaport of Mongla and on through the Bay of Bengal to the primary Bangladeshi port of Chittagong in South East Bangladesh. The population of Noapara is 170,000 and its residents have a range of employment opportunities. For more detailed information on Noapara please refer to ICCCAD (2020b).

Figure 8.1A: Food expense as a percentage of total income in September 2019

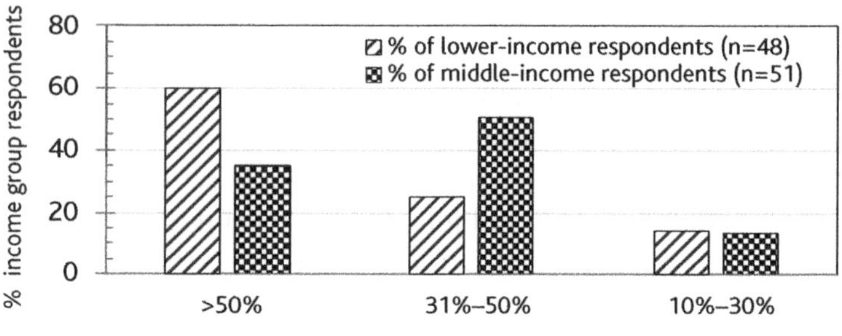

Source: authors

During the initial household survey in September 2019, it was clear that the local market was the primary outlet for sourcing food for 95 percent of respondents. Only 17 percent of respondents indicated they grew rice or vegetables. It was also apparent that food-related expenses constituted a major share of the total income of residents with nearly 60 percent of low-income and 35 percent of middle-income respondents spending over half of their total monthly income on food-related expenses (Figure 8.1A). The pre-pandemic household survey also indicated that 72 percent of the low-income and 49 percent of the middle-income respondents did not have any savings (Figure 8.1B). About 96 percent of survey respondents in Noapara indicated that they have at least three meals, however, consumption of nutritious food (for example meat, fruit, and vegetables) is less frequent among the low-income respondents compared to their middle-income counterparts.

COVID-19 lockdown's impact on food security and coping strategies

This section describes the changes in the food security situation in Noapara due to the COVID-19-induced lockdown and

Figure 8.1B: Saving status of survey respondents from Noapara in September 2019

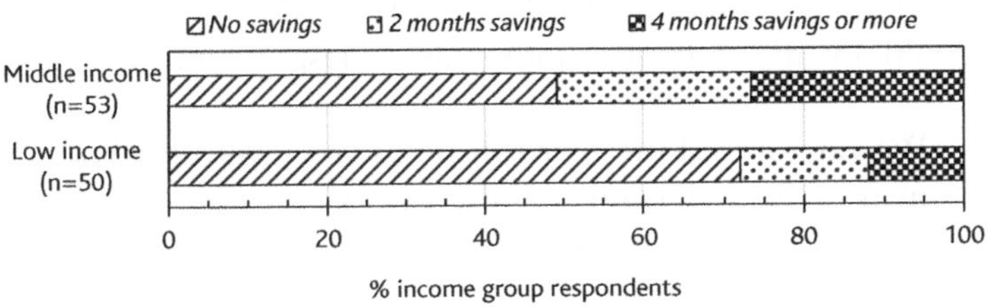

Source: authors

the coping strategies employed by the residents. The impact of the pandemic on livelihoods has been 'a disastrous situation for people from all spheres of life', according to a community leader and snack-shop owner in an informal settlement adjacent to the railway tracks in Noapara. Most interviewees reported a 75 percent to 100 percent loss of income. The severe and almost complete loss of daily income as a result of the nine-week lockdown has had a serious impact on the purchasing capacity of residents (even those described as middle class, with the exception of those who have a guaranteed income from the state or non-governmental organizations), and consequently on the quantity and quality of food being consumed. The majority of residents in Noapara lack adequate savings which explains the reported severe economic hardship after the first month of lockdown (Figure 8.1B). A female informal settlement resident from Noapara expressed her situation:

We are consuming less food in both quantity and quality. Now I cook less rice than before. Sometimes we can manage [to purchase] vegetables or spinach. As foods are dependent on our income, and I am not doing any work – so our family is dependent on the small earnings of my son.

Respondents also indicated that they had curtailed the proportion of nutritious food consumed, especially animal protein items such as meat, milk, and poultry products because they could not afford them. Another female respondent explained:

> We can't afford meat or fish nowadays. We can hardly manage [to purchase] eggs each week. We collect arum spinach from places around us and try to buy vegetables that are cheap.

Informal food providers, including street vendors and vegetable/fruit peddlers (who usually go from door to door), play an essential role in the food system of Noapara. The strict lockdown meant shutting down these businesses, resulting in not only the loss of livelihood for the owners, but also limiting access to food.

Several forms of coping strategies were identified. These included: storing food immediately before and during the first month of the lockdown (at the most, enough for one month), skipping meals or curtailing their consumption, relying on cheap starchy staples, increasing the share of total expenditure allocated to food, accessing food relief or lastly, taking loans from neighbors, friends, or loan sharks during the second month of lockdown. Rahman et al (2020) also observed similar patterns during COVID-19 in large urban informal settlements and rural areas in Bangladesh.

To limit the effects of the emerging crisis, the local government and several private donors provided food relief parcels containing rice, potato, lentils, cooking oil, onions, and soap to vulnerable groups during the lockdown. Although this support was useful, it did not reach everyone in need. From interviews with (lower) middle-income households (including small businesses) without guaranteed income, it was apparent that they were suffering as much as, if not more than low-income households in informal settlements because they could reach out for and did not qualify for food relief or social safety net programs. This may lead to middle-income households suffering from hidden or invisible food insecurity. During the pandemic, interviewees also reported taking loans from their friends and neighbors, which substantiates the importance of social capital in small cities to cope with crises.

Conclusion

To create socially inclusive, economically equitable, and environmentally sustainable cities requires a closer, comprehensive look at where people live in the world. Small, urbanizing cities are often overlooked in academic and policy research despite residents who are struggling and trying to make do with very few resources. While strategies adopted by low-income households in Noapara to cope with the lockdown-induced food insecurity were similar to those in large cities, the study also observed a set of dissimilarities between the two types of cities. Residents in small cities typically have fewer options and diversity for procuring food compared with residents of larger ones. In large cities, there is more retail competition as well as cheaper options to procure food. Respondents of this study did not report any negative coping strategies (for example distress sale of assets) during the lockdown, while this was observed in informal settlements in Dhaka (Taylor, 2020). Lastly, local government officials in small cities may have limited capacity and financial resources compared to large cities, yet the greater proximity enables local governments in these cities to act promptly and decisively during the lockdown (Ruszczyk et al, 2020). In the coming months and years, research and policy formulation need to address the relationship between structural inequality, food security, food systems, and urban sustainability. Understanding this relationship is crucial because urban poverty and food insecurity are clearly inter-related.

Acknowledgments

Our sincere thanks to Professor Louise Bracken and Professor Julian Williams from Durham University, and Mr. Istiakh Ahmed, Ms. Maheen Khan and Ms. Sumaiya Binte Selim Sudha from ICCCAD for their support throughout the research project. Funding for this work was provided by the GCRF Living Deltas Research Hub NE/S008926/1. This book chapter is also based on data collected from a 2019-2021 research project funded by the Centre for Sustainable, Healthy and Learning Cities and Neighbourhoods (SHLC)'s Capacity Development Acceleration Fund at University of Glasgow.

References

Despard, M., Grinstein-Weiss, M., Chun, Y. and Roll, S. (2020) 'Covid-19 job and income loss leading to more hunger and financial hardship'. Brookings. www.brookings.edu/blog/up-front/2020/07/13/covid-19-job-and-income-loss-leading-to-more-hunger-and-financial-hardship/

Directorate General of Health Services (DGHS) (2020) Corona COVID-19 virus dashboard 2020. http://103.247.238.81/webportal/pages/covid19.php

International Centre for Climate Change and Development (ICCCAD) (2020a) *Liveable regional cities in Bangladesh project*. www.icccad.net/programmes/resilient-livelihood/liveable-regional-cities-in-bangladesh/

International Centre for Climate Change and Development (ICCCAD) (2020b) *Noapara dissemination brief: 'liveable regional cities in Bangladesh' project*, June. www.icccad.net/wp-content/uploads/2020/06/Noapara-Dissemination-Brief-June-2020.pdf

Lawrence, F. (2020) 'UK hunger crisis: 1.5m people go whole day without food'. *The Guardian*, April 11. www.theguardian.com/society/2020/apr/11/uk-hunger-crisis-15m-people-go-whole-day-without-food

Mackay, H. (2019) 'Food sources and access strategies in Ugandan secondary cities: an intersectional analysis'. *Environment and Urbanization*, 31(2): 375–96.

Rahman, F. and Ruszczyk, H.A. (2020) 'Coronavirus: how lockdown exposed food insecurity in a small Bangladeshi city'. *The Conversation*, July 16. https://theconversation.com/coronavirus-how-lockdown-exposed-food-insecurity-in-a-small-bangladeshi-city-140684

Rahman, H.Z., Das, N., Matin, I., Wazed, M.A., Ahmed, S., Jahan N. and Zillur, U. (2020) *Livelihoods, coping and support during COVID-19 crisis*. PPRC-BIGD Response Research, Power and Participation, Research Centre and BRAC Institute of Governance and Development. https://bigd.bracu.ac.bd/wp-content/uploads/2020/05/PPRC-BIGD-Final-April-Survey-Report.pdf

Ruszczyk, H.A., Nugraha, E. and de Villiers, I. (2021) (eds) *Overlooked Cities: Power, Politics and Knowledge Beyond the Urban South*. New York: Routledge.

Ruszczyk, H.A., Rahman M.F., Bracken, L.J. and Selim, S. (2020) 'Contextualising COVID-19 pandemic's impact on food security in two small cities of Bangladesh'. *Environment and Urbanization*, 33(1): 239–54. DOI: 10.1177/09562478209655156/ ID: EAU-20-0134.R1

Satterthwaite, D. (2017) 'The impact of urban development on risk in sub-Saharan Africa's cities with a focus on small and intermediate urban centers'. *International Journal of Disaster Risk Reduction*, 26, 16–23. http://dx.doi.org/10.1016/j.ijdrr.2017.09.025

Tacoli, C. (2019) 'Editorial: the urbanization of food insecurity and malnutrition'. *Environment and Urbanization*, 31(2): 371–4.

Taylor, J. (2020) 'How Dhaka's urban poor are dealing with COVID-19' International Institute for Environment and Development (IIED) Blog, July 1. Retrieved from: www.iied.org/how-dhakas-urban-poor-are-dealing-covid-19

How Governments' Response to the Pandemic Exacerbate Gender Inequalities in Belarus and Ukraine: Comparative Analysis of Minsk and Kyiv Cases

Olga Matveieva and Vasil Navumau

Introduction

COVID-19 has had a devastating impact on urban life, with governments choosing various measures to mitigate its consequences. During the first wave of the pandemic, some countries, such as Ukraine, introduced a lockdown, closing airports and public places, and encouraging its citizens to quarantine. Others, like Belarus, preferred a 'laissez-faire' approach, ignoring COVID-19 while comparing it to the seasonal flu. This chapter analyzes the gender-related consequences of these nations' differing approaches to containing the pandemic in their respective capital cities, Kyiv and Minsk. We consider how measures implemented in the two capitals influenced both men and women during the initial phase of the pandemic (March–July, 2020).

In the first part of the chapter, we discuss the two different national policies to deal with the pandemic's consequences. We also conducted polls in Kyiv and Minsk and semi-structured, in-depth Skype interviews with eight female professionals, four in each country (politician, gender activist, feminist activist in both countries, and 'essential workers': in Belarus, a medical professional, and in Ukraine, a teacher). Questionnaires contained ten questions: the topics were chosen, proceeding from the preliminary polls, and launched via Google forms. We asked female professionals about the major problems they faced because of measures introduced by the authorities to mitigate the effects of COVID-19 (overall there were 16 questions, 93 possible answers). Via deductive reasoning, we identified the following topics: efficacy of the governments' efforts, economic pressure, an increase in household duties, psychological problems, and domestic violence. We concentrated on domestic violence as the most pressing theme. Based on the polls, we suggested the interviewees consider whether activism could be one way out of these difficult situations.

The differences between the policies in Minsk and Kyiv

Belarus, unlike neighboring countries, introduced virtually no restrictions to contain the spread of COVID-19: neither quarantine nor self-isolation were mandatory (Boguslavska, 2020). Only citizens coming from abroad were obliged to self-isolate; however, borders remained open. President Lukashenko called the pandemic 'nothing but psychosis' and suggested citizens protect themselves by engaging in sports or drinking alcohol (Hodosok, 2020). Amid the alarming news from other European countries, Minsk residents isolated themselves voluntarily, companies allowed employees to work remotely, and shops and cafés suspended their activities. This denial of the pandemic as a global threat was justified as necessary to maintain economic performance (Boguslavska, 2020). Hence, municipal authorities left the doors of educational institutions, trade centers, and other places of social activity open. This maintained the proper functioning of institutions, secured employment, and ensured a relatively stable economic situation. Still, this 'laissez-faire approach' became one of the reasons Lukashenko lost popularity ahead of the presidential elections and faced mass protests demanding him to resign (Nasha Niva, 2020b).

The situation in Kyiv (Ukraine) was completely different. Ukraine became one of the first countries in Europe to implement tough measures to counter COVID-19. In March 2020, municipalities introduced strict quarantine policies: public institutions were closed, universities moved to online teaching, citizens were banned from visiting public places, and city traffic stopped. This approach was the direct opposite of the one implemented in Belarus: the Ukrainian authorities declared they were prioritizing human lives over economic performance (Zelensky, 2020), which became the subject of public controversy. The economy, significantly weakened due to previous reforms, did not withstand the challenges of the lockdown. Many private entrepreneurs declared bankruptcy, subsequently becoming dependent on government support. This stagnation led to increasing dissatisfaction with the measures to fight the pandemic and citizens' reluctance to abide by the rules.

In general, both approaches reflected national policies: the Belarusian authorities would like to remain in power by any means (hence, they are reluctant to introduce any political or economic reforms that challenge the status quo); Ukrainian authorities are trying to respond to the global challenges of the pandemic with less attention to the economic needs of urban communities.

The main problems faced by men and women during the pandemic

We conducted an internet survey (March–July 2020) via Google forms (34 respondents) to reveal typical problems faced by Minsk residents during COVID-19, with the majority (76.5 percent) of the respondents being women. This preliminary stage revealed basic problems and allowed us to fine-tune the questionnaire. The majority of women were married with children, had higher levels of education, and represented different spheres of economic activity. The labor market both in Belarus and Ukraine is segregated, with around 80 percent of females being employed within the state system (education, social care, health care). As a result, the death rate among female medical professionals was higher than in other countries (Nasha Niva, 2020a). Therefore, because of these segregated labor markets and lower salaries for state employees, women turned out to be heavily disadvantaged during the pandemic.

The 'laissez-faire' approach divided Belarusian society: half the female respondents said the pandemic did not affect their lifestyle, whereas 52.9 percent recognized they experience depression and apathy because of unpredictability and the threat of catching the disease and infecting family members. Also, as employers were reluctant to move to working from home, they had to go to work every day. As the government did not provide informational support, 41.2 percent admitted that they faced problems with self-discipline.

A survey among Kyiv respondents (a total of 85 respondents – 70.6 percent female, sharing similar social attributes with Minsk respondents), revealed other problems. The swiftness of the government's decisions (strict quarantine and self-isolation) provided Kyiv's citizens protection from COVID-19. The representatives of 'female' professions – doctors, sellers, social-care workers, and service personnel – welcomed the introduction of the social safety nets to protect vulnerable families.

Still, the authorities did not introduce a comprehensive strategy with clear instructions to combat the pandemic in Kyiv: citizens were ordered to self-isolate, regardless of their profession, except for doctors, merchants, and civil servants. Also, economic well-being changed dramatically. One of the respondents, Ukrainian gender expert O. Ivanova concluded: 'the strong remained strong due to personal skills of resilience, the weak became even weaker and less protected, having lost the opportunity to receive help from outside'.

We summarized the main problems faced by citizens during self-isolation in Table 9.1. Further, we focus on the major problem that women in Belarus and Ukraine faced with both direct and hidden domestic violence.

Domestic violence during the pandemic

The replies of interviewees revealed that an upsurge in domestic violence occurred because people were forced to self-isolate without the ability to retain privacy.

The situation in Ukraine. The lack of information led to increased stress. The majority of men and women were neither acquainted with non-toxic ways of reducing stress nor had the necessary skills to cope with frustration. Sometimes, they resorted to alcohol, which led to a disruption of rational thought. As a result, even families with a relatively healthy atmosphere experienced cases of domestic violence (psychological pressure or assault) (UN Women, 2019).

The economic consequences of the pandemic were another problem; given that many women are dependent on men, many females suffered from aggressive behavior due to job losses or low income. Also, because of the quarantine, they had limited options for relocation (due to a lack of shelters). Hence, some women faced a difficult situation in which they had to stay in an abusive relationship, because they had nowhere to go. As one respondent said, the inconvenience of discussing domestic violence in public conversations further exacerbated complicated situations for the victims. Also, an additional factor is the lack of experts who can recognize situations in which women become victims of psychological violence.

The situation in Belarus. Social services did not record an upsurge of domestic violence because people were not enclosed within their apartments as they were in Ukraine. Still, mobile

Table 9.1: Main gender-responsive problems exposed by the pandemic and quarantine

Age	Women	Men
Up to 16	Constrained communication with peers; additional household duties; limited physical activity; home-schooling under parental pressure; domestic violence.	
17–21	Home-schooling; distanced entrance exams under parental pressure; control of private life; restriction of personal freedom; confinement of personal space; domestic violence.	
22–39	Lack of freedom of movement; constraints of habitual activity (communication, outdoor activities).	
	Increased childcare responsibilities (including education); complications of working from home; increased professional workload moved online; lack of time for rest and recovery; restricting of civic activity; peer pressure to continue being the stereotyped 'proper housewife and mother'.	Restriction of personal freedom; removal of personal boundaries; increased share of house- and childcare work (including education).
40–59	Increased risk of job loss; difficulties with a distanced format of work due to lack of technical skills, limited opportunities for employment, additional earnings; the risk of COVID-19 infection and deteriorating health and overall quality of life.	
	Social insecurity in the labor market.	Pressing obligation to continue being the stereotyped 'proper earner for the family'; less social protection.
60+	Limited income after retirement; high risk of being infected; significant complication of socialization in an increasingly digitalized reality.	

(continued)

Table 9.1: Main gender-responsive problems exposed by the pandemic and quarantine (continued)

Age	Women	Men
	Loss of social activity and break of relations due to COVID-19 related restrictions with children and grandchildren.	Decline in social activity and communication with children and grandchildren.

Source: authors

operators made the hotline for victims of domestic violence free to use. The feminist activist we interviewed stressed that around 65 percent of women had heard about increased domestic violence because of quarantine in other countries. Also, 70 percent were not satisfied with the information from the state media and preferred to look for alternative sources. As a result, 88 percent of women experienced stress and psychological tension. Activism has been recognized as one of the possible ways out.

Measures against violence. Effective state policies are necessary to prevent domestic violence, with responsibility being divided between the state, local authorities, and expert services (social services, police, control institutions). There should be zero tolerance towards this violence: every case should invoke a timely and decisive reaction. The aggressor should understand that retaliation will follow imminently. The designated specialists should monitor abusers and equip them with skills to prevent and mitigate meltdown situations (especially when children are involved). Also important, authorities should not put the responsibility for violence on family members, making it an 'internal private matter'. This is especially relevant for Ukrainian families, where the husband could be an ATO (Russia's war against Ukraine in the Donbas) veteran (Shevchenko, 2018). One purely practical solution: create of a system of shelters with the specific addresses remaining unknown to abusers.

Activism

Belarus is a consolidated authoritarian regime, where illiberal practices are rooted in everyday life and reproduced at the institutional level. This is especially typical for universities and medical institutions, hierarchical structures where the employees (mostly women) lack the ability to participate in decision-making, and activism is subject to punishment and repression. Still, 10 percent of Belarusian women claimed that they joined voluntary organizations to combat COVID-19. This determination to solve these challenges with their own hands led women to become the cornerstone of mass protest against violence in Belarus. Relying on networks of solidarity, built between activists and female professionals, women formed the backbone of 2020's revolution-in-the-making.

A gender activist stressed that activism is crucial for overcoming the harmful consequences of the pandemic because all meaningful initiatives, as a rule, start when someone opens up a public discussion about the topic, which has been heretofore silenced. When somebody supports the deliberation, certain taboos are lifted and people start looking for a solution to problems which were previously a gray area. Hence, it is important that everyone starts to individually contribute to discussions about domestic violence in Ukraine and Belarus. Still, the establishment of structured, domestic violence response systems in both countries should be a top priority, because currently this topic is dismissed as a private issue. Creating frameworks within which personal activity can be channeled is the responsibility of the state, which has a host of experts at its disposal.

Conclusion

Pandemics, like any disaster, challenge state response systems and unveil their weaknesses. As our findings from the first wave of the COVID-19 pandemic shows, the disease revealed serious problems in anti-contagion policies in both Ukraine and Belarus.

In Minsk, the social security system was not aligned to the needs of citizens and hence, was not prepared for the new challenge. Belarusians were unable to raise their concerns about the problems they faced, which eventually led to protests against the status quo. The Belarusian authorities did not recognize the threat of the pandemic: they neither introduced quarantine nor provided reliable information on necessary precaution measures. Although sharp increases in domestic violence were not registered, many women risked being infected; due to the stratification of the Belarusian labor force, women turned out to be at the forefront of struggle against the pandemic. Also, being 'traditionally' employed in low-income jobs, they became more vulnerable to being fired and thus becoming more dependent on men.

In Kyiv, the policy of containing the pandemic was expected to be 'citizen-centered'. In practice, it was implemented without consideration of gender- and age-related needs. Also, authorities suggested few measures for coping with COVID-19, besides strict self-isolation. This exacerbated serious problems in communities such as concealed and direct forms of domestic violence. Neither of the approaches implemented in Kyiv and Minsk has been successful enough to deal with the gender-specific issues faced by women in these two capital cities. It is a point of further discussion whether some 'hybrid' package of measures would be more effective: that is, without lockdown (which exacerbates the problem of domestic violence), but with a broadly effective information campaign on how to deal with the pandemic. The Belarusian case is especially problematic because the levels of trust towards authorities are quite low. The pandemic and Kyiv's quarantine regime revealed latent social problems that need to be corrected via age- and gender-responsive policies focused on providing wider opportunities for employment, social activism, and individual activities during the pandemic. The main policy-related lessons from these case studies are as follows:

- Informational: awareness-raising campaigns on the current situation within the communities with comprehensive information on morbidity dynamics, opportunities for getting help, protection of self and others, and countermeasures. Also, general advice on maintaining public and economic order, to mitigate consequences for the urban socio-economic system would be useful.
- Financial: maintenance of confidence among banks' depositors, securing the stability of prices, allocation of funds for an emergency pandemic response, providing health and social packages, subsidizing communities, supporting businesses, and ensuring continuous supply and services would all be useful in supporting citizens during a pandemic.
- Organizational: developing focused and cost-efficient measures against the spread of COVID-19 to reduce budget expenditures via focused intersectoral cooperation. This includes strategies for protecting key economic sectors and vulnerable groups (women), as well as developing strategies for 'businesses optimization' (allowing a flexible schedule, moving working processes online, partial relocation of jobs at home, ensuring social distance and safe conditions in workplaces, aligning methods for better coordination and customization, based on gender-related needs). Finally, promoting civic engagement for the provision of services and business opportunities.

Consequently, the pandemic could be an opportunity for cities to reconsider habitual practices, protocols, strategies, and programs to create a more effective and citizen-oriented public services system. This system, based on shared knowledge and national best practices of countries which succeeded in containing the pandemic, should be resilient to the second wave of COVID-19 and be more responsive to other global challenges.

References

Boguslavska, A. (2020) 'Why Belarus is not taking tough measures in the fight against coronavirus'. *Deutsche Welle*, March 30. Retrieved from: www.dw.com/ru/почему-в-беларуси-не-принимают-жестких-мер-в-борьбе-с-коронавирусом/a-52953465

Hodosok, V. (2020) '"The tractor will cure everyone". How to protect yourself from the coronavirus: Alexander Lukashenko's advice'. *Medusa*, Minsk, Belarus, March 17. Retrieved from: https://meduza.io/shapito/2020/03/17/traktor-vylechit-vseh

Nasha Niva (2020a) 'Guardian: Head of Belarus denies coronavirus, and people raise funds by crowdfunding'. Minsk, Belarus, April 18. Retrieved from: https://nn.by/?c=ar&i=250264&lang=ru

Nasha Niva (2020b) 'Ministry of Health of Belarus did not publish information on deaths caused by coronavirus but reported to UN. Data is shocking'. Minsk, Belarus, June 9. Retrieved from: https://m.nashaniva.by/articles/258542

Shevchenko, M. (2018) 'Second front: how ATO veterans aggravated the problem of domestic violence'. *Vesti*, Kyiv, Ukraine, May 3. Retrieved from: https://vesti.ua/strana/287712-vtoroj-front-kak-veterany-ato-obostrili-problemu-domashneho-nasilija

UN Women (2019) 'Left behind no more: UN women addresses inequalities women face in Ukraine'. February 5. Retrieved from: https://eca.unwomen.org/en/digital-library/multimedia/2019/02/un-women-addresses-inequalities-women-face-in-ukraine

Zelensky, V. (2020) 'Address by President Volodymyr Zelenskyy on measures to counter the spread of coronavirus in Ukraine'. *Office of the President of Ukraine*, Kyiv, Ukraine, March 13. Retrieved from: www.president.gov.ua/en/news/zvernennya-prezidenta-volodimira-zelenskogo-shodo-zahodiv-z-60161

TEN

Infrastructure Inequality and Privileged Capacity to Transform Everyday Life in COVID-19 South Africa

Charlotte Lemanski and Jiska de Groot

Introduction

This chapter, written in the midst of the ongoing COVID-19 pandemic, responds directly to its potential to deepen existing inequalities.[1] Using the example of South Africa, we highlight how COVID-19 exacerbates existing inequalities in access to infrastructure. This chapter was initially written in April 2020 (with minor updates in September 2020), in the early stages of South Africa's lockdown response to the global pandemic. The chapter has two core arguments; first, that human capacity to adhere to public health advice is privileged; and second, that global public health advice requires local contextualization.

Since December 2019 the COVID-19 virus has spread rapidly around the world, causing human fatalities, destabilizing economies, and severely restricting population movement through lockdown, social distancing, and travel restrictions. While the virus's origins are presently traced to China, this is inherently a *global* virus; not merely in terms of epidemiological geographic spread, but also the impacts across the world's social, political, and economic landscapes. However, as this chapter demonstrates, those impacts are unevenly distributed, not just between countries with differing capacity to provide, for example, health care and socio-economic support packages, but also within countries, where pre-existing inequalities are accentuated by public health advice framed by Euro-Asian contexts.

Specifically, global approaches that are directed by what is feasible in high-income countries with strong governments overlook significant divergences in the global capacity of governments, the physical and financial infrastructure of societies, alongside inequalities in citizens' ability to follow government advice to keep themselves 'safe'. This chapter identifies inequalities in the capacity of South Africa's population to comply with lockdowns and social distancing requirements, and demonstrates how COVID-19 highlights and exacerbates existing inequalities.

A global virus in the Global South

COVID-19 is a global virus, but the impact is uneven. Because it was initially concentrated in Asia, Europe, and the US, global public health responses are heavily informed by the societal structures and lifestyles of countries with high incomes and tax bases (for example Western Europe, US, Singapore) and where extreme state surveillance is common (for example China, South Korea). Globally, two non-pharmaceutical interventions have been implemented to reduce transmission rates: mitigation, and suppression. *Mitigation* aims to slow the epidemic's spread, for example through temporary lockdowns, including closing schools, cafés/restaurants, and other non-essential businesses. Many regions and countries enforced complete prohibitions on leaving home other than for essential outings (for example Hubei province, Italy, Spain, South Africa). The second strategy, *suppression*, aims to reverse the epidemic's growth by reducing secondary cases, for example via social distancing (physical avoidance of non-household members), limiting crowds, and practicing good hygiene.

While these measures, extensively promoted through social media, television, radio, public health campaigns, and government briefings/speeches, are designed to reduce transmission of the disease, they also have socio-economic implications. These implications are not captured by epidemic modeling, despite public health recognition that 'the most vulnerable groups [are] particularly those living in informal habitats and depending on informal livelihoods in the global south' (Corburn et al, 2020). Using the example of South Africa, we reveal how inequalities in access to infrastructure may exacerbate existing vulnerabilities and/or create new ones.

Privileged capacity to comply

South Africa's virus and government response

Once COVID-19 was detected in South Africa, the government responded rapidly, employing mitigation-based public health strategies seen elsewhere. Following the first confirmed case on March 5, 2020, in a patient recently returned from Italy, on March 15 (when 51 people were infected but no deaths were reported), President Cyril Ramaphosa announced a national state of disaster and commenced school closures, travel bans, and restrictions on public gatherings. One week later, the president announced a complete lockdown for 21 days, starting on March 26, 2020, when there were 927 confirmed cases and no deaths reported. This was later extended by two weeks to April 30 (that is, a five-week lockdown in total). During lockdown, people were allowed outside only for essential activities (groceries and medical outings), enforced by the military and police.

As lockdown ended, the government introduced the COVID-19 alert system to manage the shift from mitigation towards suppression. The alert system has five levels that gradually ease population restrictions, and levels are changed according to infection levels and health-sector capacity. After five weeks of full lockdown on level 5, lockdown was eased to level 4 on May 1, 2020, which allowed some essential economic sectors to operate, but lockdown remained the norm. On June 1, 2020, the country entered level 3, progressing to level 2 on August 18, 2020, and level 1 on September 21, 2020, allowing increased social activities, albeit with physical distancing required. As of September 1, 2020 there were 727,595 confirmed cases and 19,465 deaths (South African Government, 2020).

The initial March 2020 lockdown received wide public support as a necessary strategy to prevent the spread of COVID-19 and allow the state to prepare. However, the severe impacts of lockdown on the poor (where risk of starvation may be greater than risk of death due to COVID-19), raised doubt about the appropriateness of extreme lockdown (the mitigation strategy) for the South African context. Specifically, these are the inability of the urban poor to comply with lockdown by remaining 'indoors' when many lack formal shelter, the impossibility of social distancing in overcrowded high-density settlements, and the impacts of overlooking the informal food sector. The capacity of individuals to comply with government regulations is highly differentiated and reveals significant inequalities that pre-date the pandemic (see also Parker and de Kadt, Volume Two). In the next section, we highlight these inequalities, focusing specifically on the urban poor's capacity to comply with physical lockdowns and social distancing.

The privilege of 'choosing' to follow public health recommendations

Two core COVID-19 public health recommendations in South Africa are social distancing and lockdown (mask-wearing appeared later). Both require citizens to change their behavior.

We explore the assumptions inherent in each recommendation, for example regarding the practicality of infrequent shopping, and the accommodation size required to distance from others and remain indoors. These assumptions are hardly surprising given that the WHO recommendations initially emerged in countries/cities with well-developed physical and financial infrastructure networks. However, in assuming a universal capacity to comply with measures, these public health recommendations effectively ignore the prospect that compliance, far from being a choice, is impossible for some. The highest concentrations of COVID-19 infections are in low-income, densely populated, and overcrowded urban settlements where people cannot withdraw from social interactions in a single home, work remotely, buy large quantities of supplies to avoid regular shopping trips, or drive alone to secure supplies.

While recognizing that the South African government is following international 'best practice' in an extremely challenging context, we argue that public health advice tailored to local contexts is urgently required. In this chapter we reveal how a short-term pandemic highlights long-term inequalities.

Social distancing and social grants

The president's lockdown speech demanded that "everyone must do everything within their means to avoid contact with other people" (Ramaphosa, 2020). We use the example of accessing social grants to highlight the impossibility of social distancing for low-income urban dwellers. Over 17 million South Africans, one in five, depend on the government's social welfare grants (StatsSA, 2018), collected in person (due to low banking levels among the poor) at the beginning of the month. With lockdown commencing on March 26, 2020, grant payments were moved forward. Consequently social grant beneficiaries flocked to post offices, ATMs, and retail stores on and March 30 and 31, 2020 when the elderly and disability grants were available, and on April 1 for other social grants. This required beneficiaries, disproportionately highly vulnerable to COVID-19 fatality (that is, the elderly, the disabled) to expose themselves to the virus by standing in slow-moving queues for hours. While in some areas social distancing was observed, in areas with high building density and limited open space, people were in tightly packed queues. Grant recipients were also competing with those stocking up on lockdown groceries, and the media reported soldiers using violence (including rubber bullets and whips) to enforce social distancing among low-income urban dwellers queuing for food (*New York Post*, 2020). The impossibility of maintaining social distancing in this situation highlighted the limitations of the government's initial advice, which was not tailored to the practical living conditions of most urban South Africans.

Overcrowded housing in lockdown

South Africa had one of the strictest lockdowns, lasting five weeks during the spring of 2020. However, the capacity of its citizens to comply was highly unequal. Due to apartheid legacies, there is significant demographic and spatial disparity in the density and occupancy rates of urban housing. In Cape Town for example, low-density suburbs where large houses with spacious gardens accommodate middle-class nuclear families contrast with overcrowded high-density settlements on the city's periphery, where multi-generational households reside in cramped houses and shacks, cheek-by-jowl with other similarly-high occupancy housing structures (Turok, 2001). Consequently, the ability to remain indoors and to socially distance from neighbors is highly uneven. Approximately half of South Africa's population lives in low-income housing, whether in informal settlements (13.1 percent of South African households), state-subsidized housing settlements (13.6 percent), or townships (24.4 percent) (StatsSA, 2018). In all these settlements, a significant proportion of households live in (backyard) shacks that share perimeter walls built from brick, zinc, and corrugated iron (Lemanski, 2009). Not only are neighboring structures too close to satisfy social distancing requirements, but staying indoors would risk exposure to inhumane temperatures (as non-brick materials magnify outdoor temperatures) where frequently up to eight people live in one-room structures (Lemanski, 2009). It was therefore evident that remaining indoors for five weeks and maintaining social distance from other households was impossible. Consequently, the blanket government advice demonstrated absent official recognition of the realities of everyday life for South Africa's urban poor.

We do not contest the benefits of lockdown in curbing the pandemic in South Africa (Lippi et al, 2020). What we question is the overly simplistic nature of the global health advice related to lockdown. In fact, the World Health Organization (WHO) (2020) highlights the health risks of overcrowding, stating that 'inadequate shelter and overcrowding are major factors in the transmission of diseases with epidemic potential' (see also Volume 2). Consequently, the divergence between government health advice and the everyday lived realities in urban South Africa highlights how the capacity to respond to public health advice is highly differentiated and often privileged. Furthermore, there is a risk that those unable to adhere to public health recommendations are demonized for 'refusing' to comply.

Food security in lockdown

In the initial lockdown, food security was severely threatened by the prohibition of informal food vending. In urban South Africa, low-income households utilize roadside informal traders and small-scale spaza shops[2] spatially dispersed throughout settlements for daily shopping, supplemented by weekly/monthly trips to distant supermarkets (Smit et al, 2015). The informal food sector is therefore essential for low-income households to comply with lockdown. In the initial lockdown, informal food vendors were prohibited, while formal outlets, such as supermarkets and food delivery companies, were permitted. For wealthier households, typically reliant on chain supermarkets, this was 'business as usual'. For low-income households this was a hugely problematic aspect of lockdown, particularly as it coincided with the cash-lean 'hungry season' end of the month/week. While supermarkets have successfully penetrated many low-income areas, they are frequently incompatible with the consumption and food security strategies of poor households (for example the lack of electricity to refrigerate bulk items), and they typically require low-income households to walk long distances and/or pay for transport, both of which are problematic in lockdown.

After significant criticism, a small minority of registered informal vendors (registered spaza shops) were allowed to operate on April 2, 2020 (seven days into lockdown) under strict regulation (Independent Online (IOL), 2020). And on April 6, all vendors of uncooked food items were allowed to operate, subject to increased safety regulations and pending temporary municipal permits. While acknowledging the government's rapid U-turn on informal food vendors, their initial closure reveals the reliance of South Africa's government on global public health advice not tailored to local contexts.

Conclusion

This chapter responds to the potential of the COVID-19 pandemic to deepen existing inequalities. We focus on the differentiated and privileged societal capacity to transform everyday life in response to COVID-19. Using the example of South Africa, the chapter makes two core arguments.

First, that state responses to COVID-19 have not only highlighted existing inequalities, for example regarding access to basic infrastructure, but also exacerbated these inequalities, for example in distorting access to food. As the chapter demonstrates, for those living in urban poverty in South Africa, where access to basic infrastructure is limited, and where overcrowding and high density are the norm, it is frequently not possible to transform daily life in the ways required and expected by the state.

Second, that public health recommendations devised at the global scale, led by the experiences and capabilities of countries with, for example, robust tax bases, universal access to infrastructure, and strong government, require contextualization. When the COVID-19 pandemic started, governments such as South Africa's were following international 'best practice' and WHO advice. Although in principle, this is excellent advice, in practice there are significant problems with compliance for many in South Africa. While each country implements public health measures with differing intensity (for example severity of lockdown), there has been poor attention to both the needs of those most vulnerable (beyond health determinants such as age, pre-existing disease) in terms of their capacity to adhere to public health advice, as well as the capacity of different countries to support their populations in adapting to the transformations necessary for survival. The examples presented throughout this chapter indicate that broad public health advice needs adaptation to the specific empirical context of each country, and that reproductions of Euro-American/East Asian narratives are not just inadequate, they are actively harmful.

In concluding this chapter, we stress two factors that are most concerning about the (highly predictable) ways that a global pandemic exacerbates existing infrastructure inequalities. First, that public health recommendations have failed to recognize these inequalities, and to adapt advice accordingly; and second, that even in a crisis of this magnitude, the needs of the urban poor that extend well beyond this specific global pandemic remain largely overlooked. For while COVID-19 is temporary, unequal access to infrastructure is a permanent feature of urban life for many.

Notes

[1] A longer version of this chapter is published here: De Groot, J. and Lemanski, C. 2021, 'COVID-19 responses: infrastructure inequality and privileged capacity to transform everyday life in South Africa', *Environment and Urbanization*. https://doi.org/10.1177/0956247820970094

[2] A spaza shop is a small, typically unregistered, grocery store situated within residential settlements.

References

Corburn, J., Vlahov, D., Mberu, B. et al (2020) 'Slum health: arresting COVID-19 and improving well-being in urban informal settlements'. *Journal of Urban Health*, 97, 348–57. https://doi.org/10.1007/s11524-020-00438-6

Independent Online (IOL) (2020) 'Government to allow small businesses and spaza shops to operate during lockdown'. www.iol.co.za/business-report/companies/government-to-allow-small-businesses-and-spaza-shops-to-operate-during-lockdown-46370673

Lemanski, C. (2009) 'Augmented informality: South Africa's backyard dwellings as a by-product of formal housing policies'. *Habitat International*, 33(4): 472–84. https://doi.org/10.1016/j.habitatint.2009.03.002

Lippi, G., Henry, M., Bovo, C. and Sanchis-Gomar, F. (2020) 'Health risks and potential remedies during prolonged lockdowns for coronavirus disease 2019 (COVID-19)'. *Diagnosis*, 7(2): 85–90. https://doi.org/10.1515/dx-2020-0041

New York Post (2020) 'South African soldiers fire rubber bullets to enforce social distancing'. https://nypost.com/2020/03/28/south-african-soldiers-fire-rubber-bullets-to-enforce-social-distancing/

Ramaphosa, C. (2020) Statement by President Cyril Ramaphosa on escalation of measures to combat COVID-19 epidemic, Union Buildings, Tswane, South Africa. www.dirco.gov.za/docs/speeches/2020/cram0323.pdf

Smit, W., de Lannoy, A., Dover, R., Lambert, E., Levitt N. and Watson, V. (2015) 'Making unhealthy places: the built environment and non-communicable diseases in Khayelitsha, Cape Town'. *Health Place*, 29(35): 29–35. DOI: 10.1016/j.healthplace.2015.06.006

South African Government (2020) COVID-19 Statistics in South Africa. https://sacoronavirus.co.za

StatsSA (2018) *General Household Survey*. www.statssa.gov.za/?p=12180

Turok, I. (2001) 'Persistent polarisation post-apartheid? Progress towards urban integration in Cape Town'. *Urban Studies*, 38(13): 2349–77. DOI:10.1080/00420980120094551

World Health Organization (WHO) (2020) 'What are the health risks related to overcrowding?' www.who.int/water_sanitation_health/emergencies/qa/emergencies_qa9/en

ELEVEN

Under Quarantine in a City Project: Stories of Fear, Family, Food, and Community

Jeremy Auerbach, Jordin Clark, and Solange Muñoz

Introduction

In countries around the world, the COVID-19 pandemic has highlighted and exacerbated health, wealth, and racial inequalities (Ku and Brantley, 2020). In the US, Black and Brown Americans are experiencing higher mortality rates from the virus, and they are more likely to experience income loss and eviction (Benfer et al, 2020). Public housing residents in the US, while less vulnerable to housing precarity and eviction, have been directly impacted by neoliberal policies, such as the defunding of US public housing infrastructure and the increase of public–private partnerships, the effects of which the pandemic has amplified (Rice, 2017). Job loss, food insecurity, and increased marginalization from the pandemic have significant downstream effects as many US public housing residents are Black, Latino, children, elderly, or disabled (United States Department of Housing and Urban Development (HUD), 2016). These moments of crises and failure reveal the politics of urban life, but also offer the potential to identify gaps within current infrastructure and provide ways to fill them. The COVID-19 pandemic is one such moment – exposing the inequities and inaccessibility inherent in current neoliberal infrastructures. At the same time, communities are resilient and adaptable, able to produce alternative infrastructures, resources, and support.

Urban studies scholars have examined urban infrastructure as a lively socio-technic system that is 'social in every aspect' (Amin, 2014: 157). Accordingly, we define infrastructure as a complex assemblage of social and technological processes that 'enables – or disables – particular kinds of action in the city' (Graham and McFarlane, 2014: 1). During the COVID-19 pandemic, many of these urban technological processes collapsed, creating an assemblage of failure that has left a devastating gap between larger infrastructural technologies and people's livelihoods and social community. Yet, through failure, urban centers enter into a process of urban becoming, which opens engrained socio-technic systems to a necessary liveliness of bottom-up infrastructural improvisation (Amin, 2014: 156–7). We contend that people, as an infrastructure, are essential architects that guide this process of urban becoming to create emergent possibilities for an alternative community infrastructure. AbdouMaliq Simone's contention that people are infrastructures focuses on the 'collaboration among residents seemingly marginalized from and immiserated by urban life' (Simone, 2004: 407). As he argues, a community's collaborative practices have the ability to forge radical openings for a communal sense of place that may be absent or reeling in a moment of emergency (Simone, 2004: 408). COVID-19 exposed and created gaps within larger systems and urban life. The everyday community practices that emerged out of these gaps showcase routes of renewed stability through which one can reimagine urban life in a pandemic era.

This chapter takes a bottom-up approach to examine how city residents in a US public housing neighborhood, the Sun Valley housing project in Denver, Colorado, reimagined their urban life in the early stages of the pandemic, which covered the period of June and July 2020. The Sun Valley public housing neighborhood is a collection of dilapidated townhomes built in the 1950s and home to 1,500 residents who form an economically impoverished yet diverse community that includes refugees and immigrants, Black and Latinx families, single-parent households, and those who are disabled or suffer from chronic health conditions, and where more than 30 languages are spoken. Currently, Sun Valley is the city's poorest neighborhood with 83 percent of the households living below the poverty line, but the neighborhood is undergoing a major redevelopment and reinvestment including the transformation of the townhomes into mixed-income apartments.

In May 2020, 17 Sun Valley households were provided with cameras to capture images of the pandemic's impact on

Figure 11.1: The original Sun Valley townhomes with the mixed-income apartments in the background

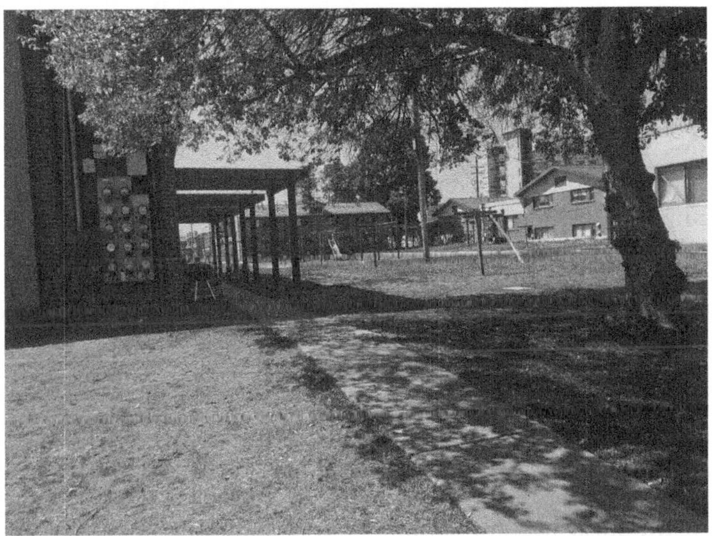

Source: authors

their environment, their daily lives, and their community. Throughout June and July of 2020, semi-structured interviews were conducted with staff of the local housing agency and residents to document their experiences and the significance of their photographs. Residents' narratives reveal the many ways the pandemic affected their lives personally and collectively and highlight how community support and resources were vital infrastructures for residents to survive and overcome public health crises. We examine these relationships through the lens of infrastructure failure and emergence to analyze how Sun Valley residents configured their daily lives and community towards alternative paths and new openings. In particular, we argue that fear, food, and family served as emergent loose ends from which residents and community organizations cultivated open connections to space and community. By taking Sun Valley residents' experiences seriously, this chapter begins to consider how these themes can serve as a framework to analyze urban infrastructure's loose ends as opportunities for a more livable city outside of moments of crisis.

Fear

As fear became a shared affect for people across the globe, the residents of Sun Valley captured how fear manifested as a continuously altered everyday life, which required them to improvise connections between people, spaces, and activities. The fear of the virus's transmission pushed individuals and families inside their homes and away from neighbors and the community, despite open yards and spaces to play. The local primary school locked its gates and yellow caution tape was pulled around the community playgrounds. For many families, this fear of the virus was connected to other feelings of uncertainty: anxiety over the loss of income, the stress of protecting their children, and the move to online schooling. The manager of the local housing authority described how: 'We weren't seeing [the families] … some kids were allowed on the stoop in the front [of their house], but you didn't see bikes for months.'

Lack of information about the virus initially created distrust, particularly among parents trying to keep their children away from others. Elena, a single mother, kept her child 'locked in the house', explaining that '[her daughter] doesn't understand that I'm just trying to … keep the distance from everybody so nobody in our family gets sick'. Fear and anxiety climaxed after the shooting and death of a resident which stemmed from an argument between families about social distancing. The institutional failures inhered in the US COVID-19 response instilled a fear that dismantled Sun Valley residents' everyday life. In reaction to their precarity and anxiety, practices of support and expansiveness emerged through connections among families and community organizers.

Family

Even when the quarantine meant negotiating cramped and crowded spaces, finding novel things to do, and sharing limited resources, the residents of Sun Valley expanded their practices and networks of support. Parents described going to great lengths to keep their children busy and healthy, while younger family members took photos of each other and described how they spent their time together. Carla, a Cameroon refugee, shared a photo of two teenage boys wrestling on the couch. She laughingly explained, 'So [this] is what I have to deal with ever since coronavirus, I have to scream every time for [my brothers] to stop wrestling, and to clean their messes up, and to do their homework.' Abdul, who lived in a three-bedroom house with 12 other family members also shared many photos of his siblings laughing and playing both inside and outside their house. During quarantine, Abdul bonded with his siblings by sharing his love for art. Mikaela, a young single mother, discussed the companionship and support she

Figure 11.2: A Sun Valley child looks out of the window during quarantine

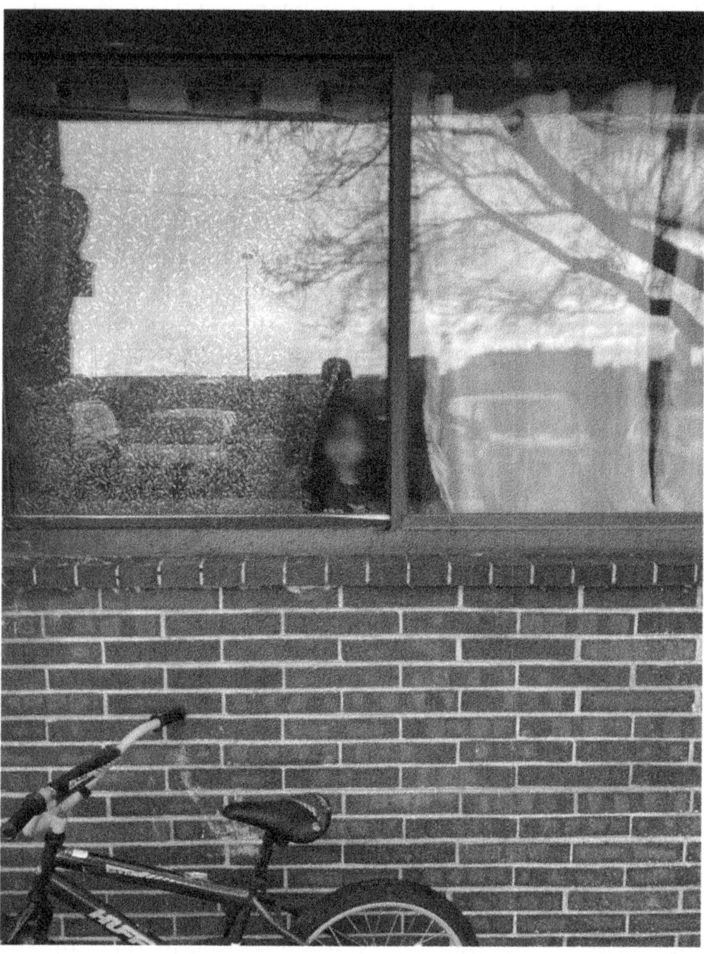

Source: authors

and her son found after her boyfriend and his daughter moved in during quarantine.

Eventually, families began to venture outdoors. One mother of four teenage boys documented the first time they went out, taking several photos of them riding their bikes and playing soccer in the park, while another mother documented and described the long walks she took with her son to the grocery store or along a nearby river trail. Set along Denver's clear blue skies, the photos convey a certain freedom and expansiveness after weeks of being indoors. Often described in detail, these acts of care and play are illustrative of the ways in which family members relied on each other and bonded as strategies to confront spatial and temporal uncertainties of the pandemic. While the pandemic necessitated that people constrict their interactions, Sun Valley's constant (re)construction of the people, spaces, and activities of family-life demonstrates the possibilities in improvising the expansion of networks and practices of support.

Food

The strengthening of the family required resources and food, which became central to community-building. As Mikaela and her partner reached a point where they 'were kind of tired of food', they began to experiment with new recipes. Several refugee families took photos of themselves preparing dishes from their home countries. Carla described in great detail a dinner she prepared:

> This is my cultural food. Anytime when I'm stressed or anything [I cook]. And these couple of months have been very stressful, very boring, and very annoying ... It is something called fufu with spinach and dried fish that I cook together ... It's a main dish in my country and it takes time to make. I made it and thought it looked good, so I took a picture of it.

She went on to talk about how much she missed her home country and the contradictions of living in the US as a Black woman. Amanda, a stay-at-home mom whose husband was furloughed once the pandemic began, took photos of herself making crab legs. She explained that that particular evening

Figure 11.3: A Sun Valley family preparing a meal together during quarantine

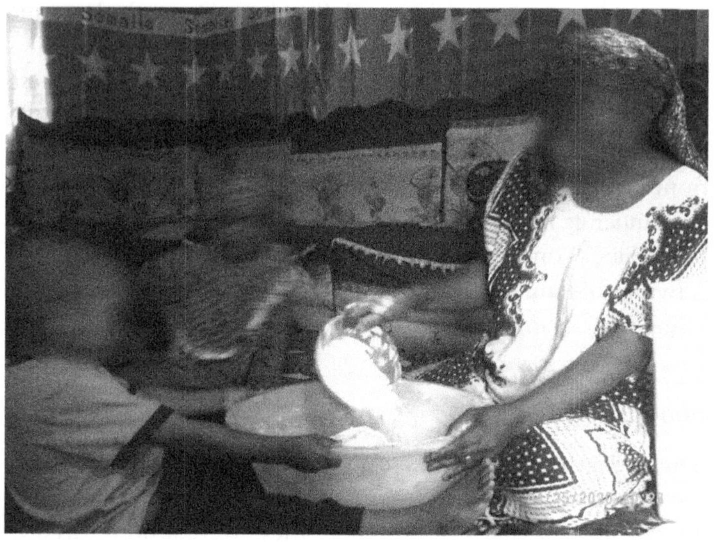

Source: authors

she was participating in a challenge in one of her Facebook groups 'to see whose crab legs came out the best-looking'. These acts of cooking allowed families to come together in their homes, but it also allowed them to connect with other people and places, in the face of COVID-19. In addition to making food, residents received seeds to grow plants and herbs, and while several residents grew plants indoors, others worked with neighbors to make small gardens in their yards. These acts of creation sow the seeds for alternative community infrastructures to sprout a nourishing sense of place replete with commitments to health, wellness, and solidarity.

Community

The emergent possibilities that residents documented actively influenced, and were influenced by the staff of the local public

Figure 11.4: A Sun Valley public housing authority staff member delivering meals to residents during quarantine

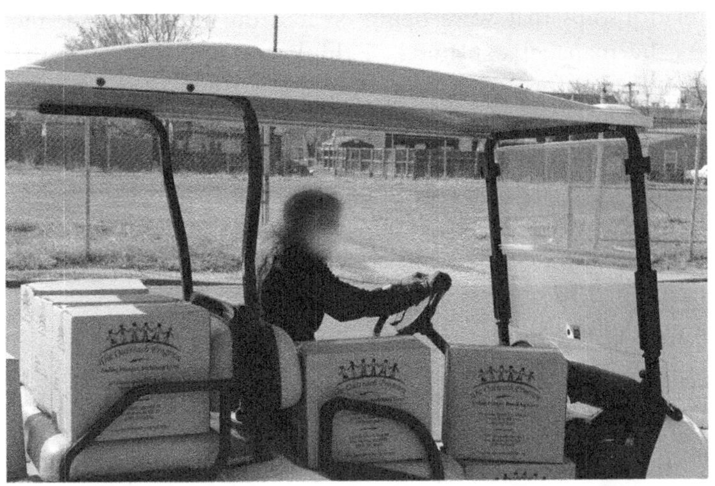

Source: authors

housing authority who are working with residents on the ongoing redevelopment project in the area. For the director and staff, the pandemic was a catalyst for investing in strategies and infrastructures that would address the individual and collective needs of the Sun Valley residents in novel ways. With residents already living in precarious and crowded conditions, staff were cognizant that the quarantine would isolate the residents further and at a moment when they would need increased support. As a result, the staff organized to bring resources and infrastructure to the residents, including food, toilet paper, and cleaning supplies. Eventually, games and activities were also delivered, so that families had things to do in their homes and outdoors. Hired by the authority as a community connector, resident Mikaela described how her relationships with her neighbors and the community changed after she delivered health and wellness kits to them. She explained, '[Before] I wouldn't even go outside, now I'm looking for residents to talk to and interact with, just to see how they are doing.' The local public housing authority also played an important role in providing some support and direction to the many new practices and relationships that were being created during the pandemic. As the manager explained, 'I think our role was to be that connection for people who didn't, at a time when we were told to not have any connections.' At the same time, she acknowledged, 'I think I learned that there were a lot more connections than I knew. I don't know if they existed before [but] I've seen a lot more connections.' We contend that some of these novel connections are emergent points of possibility developed through residents' infrastructural improvisation in a time of crisis.

Conclusion

As the fear of both COVID-19 and the impacts of its associated urban infrastructures failures spread, the residents of Sun Valley turned inward to (re)build community infrastructures through food and family. The production of these lively infrastructures offered a moment for communities to produce a shared sense of place and cultural common space (Amin, 2014: 146, 148). This chapter highlights the ways in which marginalized communities that are so used to infrastructure failure are forced to rely on individual and collective resilience to address basic needs and demands in the context of insecurity. In light of increased extreme climate events, pandemics, and failures in the political economy, Sun Valley's practices of resilience showcase what bottom-up infrastructures can emerge in urban spaces in moments of urgency, which becomes particularly salient when we consider people as an infrastructure.

This chapter draws attention to the diverse emotional, physical, and relational needs of a community, and suggests that they should be taken seriously as a prominent infrastructure for community survival and nourishment. Of course, Sun Valley is only one example of the many communities around the globe facing similar infrastructural failure. But, its lessons on how local residents fill the gaps within top-down infrastructure through a more people-centered approach can instruct larger, global infrastructural processes. Creating a community infrastructure that promotes a sense of place and cultural commons, stems from making lively infrastructures visible and acknowledging their significance as alternative and viable possibilities. Through the combination of photography and semi-structured interviews, this bottom-up methodology showcases how residents made their emerging community infrastructures, which are now visible to a global audience, and is one that can easily be adapted for other populations. Making the Sun Valley experience visible shows urban planners, scholars, and community organizations a path forward as we navigate how to center people in the development of more just infrastructures during and beyond the COVID-19 pandemic.

References

Amin, A. (2014) 'Lively infrastructure'. *Theory, Culture & Society*, 31(7–8): 137–61. https://doi.org/10.1177/0263276414548490

Benfer, E., Robinson, D.B., Butler, S., Edmonds, L., Gilman, S., Mckay, K.L., Neumann, Z., Owens, L., Steinkamp, N. and Yentel, D. (2020) 'The COVID-19 eviction crisis: an estimated 30–40 million people in America are at risk'. The Aspen Institute, August 7. Retrieved from: www.aspeninstitute.org/blog-posts/the-covid-19-eviction-crisis-an-estimated-30-40-million-people-in-america-are-at-risk/

Graham, S. and McFarlane, C. (2014) *Infrastructural Lives: Urban Infrastructure in Context*. New York: Routledge.

Ku, L. and Brantley, E. (2020) 'Widening social and health inequalities during the COVID-19 pandemic'. JAMA Health Forum, June 10. Retrieved from: https://jamanetwork.com/channels/health-forum/fullarticle/2767253

Rice, D. (2017) 'Budget caps, not rent aid, forcing HUD budget cuts'. Retrieved from: www.cbpp.org/research/housing/budget-caps-not-rent-aid-forcing-hud-budget-cuts

Simone, A. (2004) 'People as infrastructure: intersecting fragments in Johannesburg'. *Public Culture*, 16(3): 407–29. https://doi.org/10.1215/08992363-16-3-407

United States Department of Housing and Urban Development (HUD) (2016) *Resident characteristics report as of May 31, 2016.* Retrieved from: www.hud.gov/program_offices/public_indian_housing/systems/pic/50058/rcr

TWELVE

The Impacts of Socio-Spatial Inequity: COVID-19 in São Paulo

Roberto Rocco, Beatriz Kara José, Higor Carvalho, and
Luciana Royer

This chapter addresses the multidimensional impacts of the
COVID-19 pandemic on the lives of citizens of one of the
largest and most unequal metropolises in the world, São Paulo.
It is widely recognized that Brazil's response to the COVID-19
pandemic has been more than flawed, with a disproportionate
impact on poor and indigenous communities (Curtice, 2020;
The Lancet, 2020). The virulent politicization of the pandemic
set the powerful federal government, in the hands of a far-right
populist, on a collision course with the interests of federal
states and cities in Brazil. While the Brazilian president has
repeatedly denied the gravity of the pandemic, states and cities
struggled to impose partial lockdowns and to organize medical
responses, in the face of contradictory policy being enacted in
their distant capital, Brasilia. This chapter describes the structural circumstances that led São Paulo to become one of the
cities worse affected by the virus, leading to the almost complete collapse of its public health system. While COVID-19
was initially perceived as the 'great equalizer', infecting all

regardless of race or social class, it soon became apparent that marked socio-spatial inequity means the effects of the pandemic are felt differently by various socio-economic groups in the city (see Xavier, Volume 2).

In order to approach these differences from a multi-dimensional perspective, we give accounts of three life-stories under the pandemic that illustrate these issues. These short accounts outline the daily lives of three 'Paulistanos' (inhabitants of São Paulo) who must negotiate urban space and access citizens' rights in radically diverse ways. These accounts address issues of class, race, gender, political ideology, and space. The short narratives are drawn from a small pool of semi-structured interviews with citizens representative of larger categories conducted for this chapter and provide the reader with input on the several ways COVID-19 has impacted the lives of citizens from individual perspectives that nevertheless illustrate collective struggles. The main methods utilized are life-stories and discourse analysis. We briefly describe their accounts, connect them to wider trends and challenges in the city, and reflect on the issues unveiled by the pandemic and ponder the meaning of socio-spatial inequality for citizens' access to rights (for a similar approach, see Lindenberg et al, Chapter Nineteen).

Eliana S., the cleaner

Eliana is a short and stout White Brazilian woman who works as a cleaner for several middle-class households. She is 54 years old and came from Aracaju, a large city in northeast Brazil, in the 1990s, together with her former husband and three children, now adults. Eliana lives in a *favela* (slum).

The Brazilian Institute of Geography and Statistics (IBGE) estimates the number of precarious dwellings is 5.12 million, or 7.2 percent of the total number of dwellings in the country (IBGE, 2020). Most precarious dwellings are in favelas, which are characterized by high density, the absence or incompleteness of sanitation infrastructure, and precariousness of construction. Many slums have transitioned from temporary housing to permanent alternatives for many families, and their makeup has changed towards masonry houses, sometimes with more than one floor.

It is noteworthy that favelas are far from being uniform spatial units: a favela can house many different social groups simultaneously, and this is reflected in the quality of spaces. Eliana is not among the worse-off in the slum where she lives in a small rental house. Even so, her family's quarantine in a confined space and in a dense environment triggered significant transformations to Eliana's life. Eliana alone provides for a household that includes her ex-husband, who, at the bequest of her daughters was welcomed back by her, and her youngest son, aged 23. Her daughters have already left home. Their house is about 40 m^2, with two bedrooms, a living room, bathroom, and kitchen. In March 2020, with the start of the quarantine, Eliana's weekly cleaning jobs in middle-class homes were suspended. However, the three families for whom she works every week kept paying her daily rates, without which the R$800 [US$150] rent and other expenses could no longer be paid. To complement this income, she accessed the R$600 [US$112] emergency aid provided by the federal government to informal workers in March 2020.

During quarantine, her son decided to set up a food production and delivery service at home. Eliana worked with him, 'to supervise hygiene precautions', together with a young woman hired to help. To complicate matters further, her son and the newly hired assistant started dating and she also moved into the house, making the family's confinement 'unbearable' according to Eliana. Despite the lockdown, the son and his new girlfriend continued to go out locally, making Eliana extremely nervous:

It was very difficult to stay with everyone [in a small house], a struggle, having the experience of spending all day with them, maintaining the hygiene required by the quarantine, insisting that they isolate themselves, for the boy to stop going to the bar to drink, to do the proper hygiene on arrival.

In order to deal with overcrowding, Eliana chose to isolate herself in her bedroom, even taking her meals there. 'I felt helpless. I thought there wouldn't be any more jobs for me, for anyone. I stopped watching TV, it scared me to see people dying. I started to get depressed.'

In the second month of the quarantine, she called the families she used to work for, asking to go back to work – she could not stand being isolated inside her own house any more and could not bear the uncertainty of not having a job, although her income was assured for the moment. Initially, her bosses did not allow her to go back to work, assuring her she would still get paid until the quarantine was over, but she insisted. A new challenge began – getting to work while avoiding exposure to the virus as much as possible. Crowds frighten Eliana: 'I do my part, but others don't.' When São Paulo's mayor reduced the number of buses circulating – a measure allegedly taken to encourage isolation – people were angry, arguing that buses had become even more packed than usual. According to Eliana, if someone coughs or sneezes on the bus, other passengers try to throw them out. Eliana has a hard time differentiating between the actions of different levels of government but realizes that there is a dispute between them. 'The reduction of buses by the mayor was not right, but the new measures, such as the use of masks, and the emergency aid, were good (...) there has never been a president who provided such assistance (...) but this money comes from us, from our taxes, nothing is free.' Although he was initially opposed to it, the emergency aid helped improve the president's popularity: 'For Bolsonaro, it was a victory. On the bus, people say he'll win the next election.'

Givanildo P., the community organizer

Givanildo is a 20-year-old, bespectacled, short and slim young man, impeccably dressed in khaki trousers and polo shirt. It would be difficult to classify Givanildo's ethnicity, but in North America he would be classified as 'Latino'. He speaks with a mild north-eastern accent and gives his interview via Zoom, sitting in his car outside Paraisópolis Community Center. Paraisópolis is the biggest slum in São Paulo, with more than 100,000 inhabitants living in 118 hectares (IBGE, 2010). It is also the densest neighborhood in the country, with 45,000 people per square kilometer (Oliveira, 2016), making it impossible to practice 'social distancing'. Although Paraisópolis is widely recognized as a *favela* and has all the attributes of one, its citizens never refer to it as such, preferring instead to call it 'the community'. Only 25 percent of Paraisópolis inhabitants have access to sanitation, half the streets are unpaved, and 60 percent of households taps into the energy grid illegally (Oliveira, 2016). Although more than 90 percent of households have access to running water, water provision is defective and has prompted the state government to provide 2,400 household water reservoirs to improve regular access during the pandemic (Souza, 2020).

Givanildo is a community leader and 'cultural producer' and is one of the leaders of the Paraisópolis taskforce against COVID-19. He helped create and coordinate the pandemic response model known as 'Street Presidents', in which a community representative is directly responsible for monitoring the well-being of 50 families, relaying detailed information to the community organizers. The community also hired their own ambulances and trained citizens to act as paramedics in cases of emergency. The community's efforts to contain the virus brought the morbidity rate to 21.7/100,000 inhabitants in May 2020. These numbers were below 30.6 found in the surrounding high-income neighborhood of Vila Andrade and much lower than the city's rate of 56.2 (Instituto Polis, 2020). This situation changed dramatically later in the pandemic, from 16 deaths per 1,000 inhabitants in May 2020 to 54 deaths per 1,000 inhabitants in August 2020. 'For the public health doctor and researcher at the Polis Institute, Jorge Kayano, there was an exhaustion of community actions over the months. "All the measures that have been adopted end up being exhausted over time because they are no longer able to contain the population inside their homes hoping to end the pandemic," he points out' (Mello, 2020).

Givanildo came to São Paulo with his family from the impoverished north-eastern Brazilian State of Paraíba when he was 12. He says Paraisópolis welcomed the family, who initially had to live in a very precarious shack. Givanildo points out he had several advantages in comparison to slum dwellers elsewhere. He earned a scholarship for primary and secondary education and was able to enter a private university where he studies system analytics. It soon became clear to him that he ought to "pay back" the community, and he started organizing when he was still in secondary school. His latest project is a "flood sensor" that warns inhabitants of upcoming flashfloods in the low-lying parts of the slum through a smartphone app. Three years ago, Givanildo's family moved to the countryside, but he decided to stay in a small house owned by his family inside the slum. However, with the pandemic, community leaders decided to rent a house outside of the slum where they share the expenses and shelter together. They did so for safety reasons, and to be able to coordinate the community's response to the virus without the burdens of overcrowding, conflict, and irregular access to running water.

Givanildo coordinates Paraisópolis participation in the G10 Slum Summit, a network of community leaders from the ten largest slums in Brazil, which got together to improve social and economic development and participation in their communities and is now present in 13 Brazilian states (G10, 2020).

He recognizes that unemployment has skyrocketed in Paraisópolis during the quarantine but points out that the slum has a robust internal economy which "in normal times shields it from economic crises", with 16,000 small business, four bank branches, a big supermarket, and other big stores. Many Paraisópolis dwellers work in the informal economy and do not have to travel far, as many of their jobs are in Morumbi, a high-end neighborhood next to the slum.

Givanildo is politically aware and criticizes the lack of attention from local authorities to the community. He is especially critical of the discourse of "new normal", as "Brazilian *favelas* have never reached the normal. As they [the government] don't do anything for us, we have decided to help ourselves. They only remember we exist when they need our votes. So, we community organizers, have decided not to support any particular political parties". While he is not able to evaluate the support of inhabitants to the far-right president of Brazil, he says that among his team of 250 community organizers, not one supports the current president. "Bolsonaro is killing people."

Ho Y.L., the medical doctor

Ho Y.L. was born in Taiwan and came to Brazil at the age of ten. In São Paulo, she studied medicine and today, at 48, she is the chief physician of the Intensive Care Unit (ICU) at Hospital das Clínicas, considered one of the best hospitals in Latin America. The hospital is part of the Brazilian Unified Health System, known by its Portuguese acronym SUS. SUS is widely praised as a model of universal health care in the Global South (World Health Organization (WHO), 2013). Ever since Bolsonaro's election, SUS has faced underfunding and threats of privatization by the federal government, which puts an additional strain on Ho. She exudes calmness and confidence, but her fatigue after a long shift is visible in the online interview she gave us.

Ho was hired by the federal government to go to Wuhan, China, together with the Brazilian Air Force and technicians from the Ministry of Health, to repatriate 34 Brazilian nationals who were in lockdown in that city. Two weeks after her return, the first domestic case of COVID-19 was reported, and Ho saw the ICU she coordinates go from seven to 300 beds, all dedicated exclusively to patients with symptoms of COVID-19.

Ho lives alone in her own seven-room apartment, in an upper-middle-class neighborhood in the southwest side of São Paulo. Despite the favorable conditions for social isolation, she kept working at the hospital, only isolating when she contracted the virus herself. During the 14 days of isolation, Ho continued to guide her team remotely through WhatsApp messages, while still in bed. Upon recovering, she immediately returned to work. At the hospital, she witnessed the contradictions of the pandemic in Brazil. On several occasions, her medical team struggled to contact patients' family members because they had also been infected and were no longer home. Doctors noticed a pattern of overcrowding in these cases. On one occasion, the relatives of a patient forcefully asked Ho to prescribe hydroxychloroquine, following Brazil's president's recommendations on social media. "Here, we work only based on scientific evidence," she replied, in reference to the debunked conspiracy theories inexplicably repeated on TV by the country's president. Ho believes that there is a lack of awareness within the population of the gravity of the pandemic, aggravated by mixed messages from the federal government. She worries about the lack of sanitation in more vulnerable neighborhoods of the city. As for the management of the pandemic, Ho ponders that Brazil was handling the crisis well until the departure of the Minister of Health who was in conflict with the president. The latter insisted the virus was "just a little flu" (Borges, 2020). After that, state governors' protagonism became more significant in combating the pandemic. For Ho,

"COVID-19 is a disease that is here to stay, and we should learn to deal with it."

Conclusion

For Flávio Villaça, one of the greatest Brazilian urbanists:

> (…) no aspect of Brazilian society can ever be well explained without considering the enormous economic and political inequality that occurs in our society. Brazil's biggest problem is not poverty, but the inequality and injustice associated with it. (Villaça, 2011)

This inequality is inevitably reflected in socio-spatial fragmentation and segregation. This means that COVID-19 has had a heterogeneous impact on diverse groups in this gigantic metropolis, as shown in the 'Inequality Map of the City of São Paulo' (Rede Nossa São Paulo, 2020). Not surprisingly, wealthy districts are places where people can work from home and can self-isolate. These districts tend to have longer life expectancy, and are where deaths from COVID-19 grew at a much slower rate. At the other end, in districts where people have lower life expectancy, people cannot self-isolate effectively and many citizens work in the informal economy. These places, normally located in the distant eastern and southern peripheries of the city, were disproportionately impacted by the virus. Socio-spatial fragmentation in São Paulo also has a clear racial bias. 'The two districts with the highest proportion of blacks, Jardim Angela (60%) and Grajaú (57%), had the high number of COVID-19 deaths, at 507. In contrast, the two districts with the lowest proportion of blacks among their inhabitants, Alto de Pinheiros (8%) and Moema (6%), registered only 110 deaths due to the virus' (Rede Nossa São Paulo, 2020). The former neighborhoods are in the peripheries of the city, and their inhabitants must spend hours on public transportation to get to work. They also house the people who do not have the option of working from home and cannot give up working, as they live from payday to payday. The case of Eliana, with understanding bosses who were willing to pay her even if she did not come to work, was an exception. It is significant, however, that where citizens took the response to COVID-19 in their own hands, the number of deaths was considerably lower, at least initially. However, the poor living conditions of vulnerable people we have described in this chapter meant that, in the end, the pandemic caught up with Paraisópolis. Community engagement apparently had the effect of making inhabitants of Paraisópolis much better informed about how to avoid the virus, but their material conditions and the lack of supporting government action meant that no amount of community organization could shield them from the virus. This contrasts with the experience of middle- and upper-class Paulistanos, who could shelter and work from home. Finally, the political meaning of the pandemic cannot be overstated. While support for the controversial President of Brazil suffered from his botched response to the crisis, he gained popularity with the emergency aid provided to poor families. It remains to be seen how Brazilians will respond to a continuing botched response, largely based on conspiracy theories and science-avoidance.

References

Borges, A. (2020) ' "A little flu": Brazil's Bolsonaro playing down coronavirus crisis'. *Euronews*, April 10. Retrieved from: www.euronews.com/2020/04/06/a-little-flu-brazil-s-bolsonaro-playing-down-coronavirus-crisis

Curtice, K. (2020) 'Indigenous populations: left behind in the COVID-19 response'. *The Lancet*, 395(10239): 1753.

G10 (2020) *G10: Bloco de Líderes e Empreendedores de Impacto Social das Favelas*. Retrieved from: www.g10favelas.org

IBGE (Brazilian Institute of Geography and Statistics) (2010) *Aglomerados subnormais 2019: classificação preliminar e informações de saúde para enfrentamento à COVID-19.* Retrieved from: https://biblioteca.ibge.gov.br/index.php/biblioteca-catalogo?view=detalhes&id=2101717

IBGE (Brazilian Institute of Geography and Statistics) (2020) *Aglomerados Subnormais 2019: Classificação preliminar e informações de saúde para enfrentamento à COVID-19.* Retrieved from: https://biblioteca.ibge.gov.br/visualizacao/livros/liv101717_apresentacao.pdf

Instituto Polis (2020) *Paraisópolis tem melhor controle da pandemia que o município de São Paulo.* Retrieved from: https://polis.org.br/noticias/paraisopolis/

Mello, D. (2020) 'Taxa de mortalidade por COVID-19 em Paraisópolis aumenta 240%'. Agencia Brasil. Retrieved from: https://agenciabrasil.ebc.com.br/saude/noticia/2020-09/taxa-de-mortalidade-por-covid-19-em-paraisopolis-aumenta-240-0

Oliveira, N.d. (2016) 'IBGE divulga Grade Estatística e Atlas Digital do Brasil'. Retrieved from: https://agenciabrasil.ebc.com.br/economia/noticia/2016-03/ibge-divulga-grade-estatistica-e-atlas-digital-do-brasil

Rede Nossa São Paulo (2020) *Edição extraordinária do Mapa da Desigualdade indica CEP como fator de risco na pandemia.* Retrieved from: www.nossasaopaulo.org.br/2020/06/24/edicao-extraordinaria-do-mapa-da-desigualdade-indica-o-endereco-como-fator-de-risco-na-pan/

Souza, C. (2020) 'Paraisópolis ganha caixas d'água, mas moradores relatam torneira seca'. *UOL.* Retrieved from: https://noticias.uol.com.br/cotidiano/ultimas-noticias/2020/04/06/em-sp-paraisopolis-ganha-caixas-dagua-mas-nao-tem-agua-em-torneiras.htm

The Lancet (2020) 'COVID-19 in Brazil: "So what?" (Editorial)'. *The Lancet*, 395(10235): 1461. https://doi.org/10.1016/S0140-6736(20)31095-3

Villaça, F. (2011) 'Segregação urbana e desigualdade'. *Revista Estudos Avançados*, 25(71): 37–58.

World Health Organization (WHO) (2013) *Arguing for universal health coverage*. Retrieved from: www.who.int/health_financing/UHC_ENvs_BD.PDF?ua=1

PART III

Migration, Migrants, and Refugees

Liminality, Gender, and Ethnic Dynamics in Urban Space: COVID-19 and its Consequences for Young Female Migrants (YFM) in Dhaka

Ellen Bal, Lorraine Nencel, Hosna J. Shewly, and

Sanjeeb Drong

Introduction

This chapter presents the changing situation of female workers in the Ready-Made Garment industry (RMG) and the beauty parlor sector in Dhaka, the capital city of Bangladesh, as an outcome of the COVID-19-virus/crisis. Both sectors predominantly employ women. Before the pandemic, there were nearly four thousand active RMG factories in Bangladesh, employing a total of 3.5 million workers. Approximately 60 percent were female and 40 percent were male.[1] In 2009, the personal care industry was reported to employ about 100,000 women in about 2,000 registered beauty parlors, mainly in urban areas all over the country (see Grabska et al, 2015: 64). The beauty parlor sector is known for many of its employees being Garo, one of Bangladesh's 50 officially recognized indigenous minorities. The Garos, who are predominantly Christian, had a distinctive advantage in particular job opportunities in cities, such as nursing or hairdressing, which used to be regarded as polluting both by Muslims and Hindus (Bal, 2007; Raitapuro and Bal, 2016). This chapter is based on several online conversations with different partners[2] currently situated in Bangladesh, and the results of an in-depth ethnographic research project on young female migrants in Dhaka, which we carried out from March 2016 to October 2018.[3]

For more than 20 years, women's presence in the urbanscape of Dhaka increased exponentially, completely changing the face of this urban space. A recent study noted that before COVID-19, three out of every five migrants from rural areas were female, signifying a remarkable shift from the traditional male dominance in the labor force in urban areas. The job opportunities that opened up for young women in the RMG industry since the 1980s, and especially after the turn of the century in particular, are a key factor in this migration.

Pandemics are known to reproduce and exacerbate existing social inequalities present in society (Lokot and Avakyan, 2020). In this chapter, we will trace the trail of responses that COVID-19 has provoked for women working in the RMG and beauty parlor sectors. It will become clear that even though the working conditions and their positions in society differ greatly, the consequences of COVID-19 for these marginalized groups of female workers affect them in similarly harsh ways. In the early phase of the crisis, nearly all of these women lost their jobs and returned to their villages for an indeterminate amount of time, putting their livelihoods further at stake and their families in crisis. While parlors have kept their doors largely closed, the RMG sector is trying to get back to business as some canceled orders have been reinstated.

In trying to make sense of the responses and outcomes produced by COVID-19, we found that the situation in Bangladesh can be seen as a period of liminality (see also

Banerjee and Das, Volume 2). Millions of Bangladeshis are living in fundamental insecurity, experiencing a time that is different from what they were used to, while being uncertain as to what their future will bring. Pandemics, as asserted by Cangià (2020), are 'a phase which comes between past and future yet belongs neither to the past as we knew it, nor to the future as we imagined it'. They can be described as the 'pause before the new beginning' in which people 'exist outside our lives and outside of time' (Awdish, 2020). Liminality is commonly used to refer to a period of fundamental uncertainty during which existing social hierarchies are reversed or temporarily dissolved, and future outcomes once taken for granted are thrown into doubt (for example Van Gennep, 1960; Thomassen, 2009). The notion, therefore, gives us the potential to conceptualize the current situation in Bangladesh. The liminal period provoked by COVID-19 has caused shifts and interruptions in the labor market as well as in women's daily lives. We will see later how these have reinforced unequal gender relations as well as demanded both workers and management to rework and reshuffle pre-existing labor relations and daily household and livelihood routines. After a brief description of the current situation under COVID-19, we will illustrate how these changes converged to intensify the liminal conditions of young migrant workers.

Bangladesh in times of COVID-19

Bangladesh had three months to prepare for the pandemic after COVID-19 affected China in January 2020. Health experts, civil society, and others demanded effective preparation. The government, however, undertook very little preparation in order to face the crisis as it unfolded gradually. The budget allocated for crisis management got lost in utterly corrupt public-private partnerships, resulting in the highest numbers of doctors' deaths compared to other countries. Newspaper reports of fake ventilators, N-95 masks, and Personal Protective Equipment

(PPE) went viral on social media, enhancing frustration and fear among the population. The lockdown measures proclaimed in April 2020 were hardly controlled and enforced, and people barely followed social distancing rules because of various confusing messages that came from the government, religious leaders, and government health experts.

By early September 2020, Bangladesh counted a total of 325,157 cases and 4,634 deaths.[4] According to government statistics, a total of 1,704,758 tests were conducted among a population of 164,880,000 people.[5] This number was not only far below the benchmark set by the World Health Organization (WHO), but was also the lowest in South Asia.[6] (Al-Amin et al, 2020). It is worth mentioning that after Bangladesh introduced a high testing fee, the country's testing numbers fell. In a country where one in four live below the national poverty line, this fee is an obstacle for the poor to be tested for COVID-19. Daily briefings on COVID-19 stopped on August 11, 2020, as the government felt the situation had improved, and the Health Minister of Bangladesh claimed that COVID-19 would soon leave Bangladesh on its own.[7] Overall, the first wave of pandemic not only exposed the irregularities and corruption in the health sector in Bangladesh but also the government's mismanagement and lack of coordination and a tendency to conceal COVID-19-related information.

Bangladesh's economy also suffered a huge blow due to COVID-19. It has been estimated that around 15 to 20 million people, from different economic sectors, are at risk of losing their jobs due to the slowdown of trade and business.[8] The pandemic has especially affected the informal and labor-oriented sectors, including the ready-made garments industry (RMG). Contributing around three quarters of Bangladesh's total export earnings, the RMG sector is pivotal to Bangladesh's economic growth. The pandemic disrupted global supply chains, and international brands and retailers suspended $3.8 billion worth of clothing orders from Bangladesh, affecting

2.2 million workers.[9] In March 2020, export earnings were just 44.14 billion taka (€460.5 million), compared to 256.66 billion taka (€2.68 billion) in the same month in the previous year.[10] The RMG sector began to grow again during the summer of 2020, before the second wave arrived. Ready-made garment exports fell 9.69 percent in December 2020 compared to the previous year, led by an 18 percent drop in sales of woven garments.[11]

Perhaps even more worrisome were the approximately 50 million people employed in the informal sector. This sector includes not only hotel and restaurant workers and the transportation and building sectors where women are less prominent, but also domestic work, sex work, and the beauty industry, in which women and children predominate. According to the South Asian Network on Economic Modelling (SANEM), Bangladesh's poverty rate may double to 40.9 percent compared to prior to the onset of the pandemic.[12]

The lockdown measures of the government and many other employment uncertainties caused a huge outflow of workers from cities back to their home villages (see also Banerjee and Das, Volume 2). Newspaper articles highlighted the massive movement of migrant workers to villages after the announcement of lockdown. Thousands of male and female workers walked, or piled into overcrowded trucks or vans to leave the city as public transport was shut during the lockdown and factory or parlor management did not provide any alternative transportation. By June 2020, over 15 percent of Dhaka's 18 million population left the city, while 1.26 percent arrived in the city from other districts.[13] Workers' incomes in the city declined by an average of 42 percent in July 2020.

In the following section, we will take a closer look at the particular ways RMG workers and Garo beauticians have been affected by these shifts and interruptions, increasing their insecurity and intensifying the liminal conditions produced by the pandemic.

Reinforcing, reshuffling, and reworking the pre-existing present

Complying with the government-declared lockdown (when only emergency services were open), from March 26, 2020, all garments factories were closed, many without paying the workers their salaries, resulting in protests on the streets.[14] Returning to their villages was the only option open to these workers, as housing and even minimal necessities became too expensive in the city. The move, however, also put a halt to their means to earn money, interrupting their livelihoods as well as suspending their well-established social networks, which are vital if one intends to come back to work and live in this urban center (see also Brooks, Chapter 5; Minas, Volume 4).

The return to the villages has reinforced pre-existing unequal gender relations reflected in the increase in gender-based violence, as well as the increase in early marriage. Whereas previously, fake birth certificates were obtained for minors to be employed in the cities, recently it has been noted that this tactic is being used to marry off young girls under the minimum legal age of 16. With less money entering households, early marriage offers a way to lessen the economic burden.[15] While women's migration to the city did not do away with these existing forms of patriarchal power, it did give them more space to maneuver, which in some cases was abruptly brought to a halt.

A few months after COVID-19 hit Bangladesh, some kind of 'normality' returned and many people started coming back to Dhaka. One year later, however, the COVID-19 situation continues to be unstable and many of the garments workers and beauticians still find themselves without work back home in their villages. With limited labor opportunities available in the city, families seem to be reconsidering who to send, and men more than women appear to be returning. Most RMG workers who have been called back have accepted the difficult circumstances, choosing income over protecting their health and labor rights. Their return is occurring with a certain amount of reshuffling of labor standards, which had been obtained in previous years through union struggles and global pressure. Their negotiation and bargaining capacity have been reduced due to the changing circumstances of the job market. Labor rights, such as minimum wage and overtime payment, have been readjusted to what management claims to be the only way for the factories to survive. Thus, existing legislation and labor conditions have been unofficially suspended.

Although parlor workers do not enjoy the same labor rights as RMG workers, a similar tendency is found in the beauty parlor sector. While a large majority of parlors have kept their doors closed, a well-known beauty parlor reopened its doors before the Muslim festival of Eid al-Adha in the summer of 2020. Some workers were called back to take up their jobs. Customers, however, did not return in large numbers and the beauticians only received one third of their normal salaries. In anticipation of new attempts to open the doors, some Garo women remained in the city. Instead of renting housing with their family, who remained in the villages, sharing rooms with co-workers to cut down expenses is quite common. Hence a reshuffling of household dynamics can also be observed since these migrants returned. In the RMG sector too, workers opted to share rooms even more than before, in order to soften the economic burden of earning substantially less money. Local rents have been reduced and 'To let' signs can be observed across the entire city.

Finally, the existing labor relations are being reworked. In the RMG sector, senior employees are being replaced (fired, no salaries paid) by new workers (for lower salaries); men stand better chances in (re)negotiating their employment contracts and salaries than women. RMG workers are reconsidering working in the informal sector such as domestic work or street vending. Equally, Garo beauticians out of work are reworking their employment opportunities. Garos' initial entrance into the urban labor market was through domestic work, more specifically for expat communities where they were known in most cases to be treated well and respected. With the virtual disappearance of expat communities from Dhaka, Garo parlor workers are now considering working for Bengali families, which, considering the ethnic discomfort between the communities, would not have been likely in the past.

Conclusion

COVID-19 has created a liminal space in which various types of relations (work, family, ethnic, belonging to the city) are being reshuffled and interrupted. This manifests itself in the reinforcement of work-related exploitation and patriarchy. It has suspended the bargaining capacity of (young) women at work and at home, and has caused pre-existing labor, gender, and ethnic relations to be reconsidered. This liminal period has slowed down the feminization of internal migration to Dhaka which had accelerated since the turn of the 21st century, thereby momentarily at least, altering the face and organization of urban space. The entrance of young women into the labor market, and thereby urban space, allowed many of them to support their families back home, fund their siblings' education, invest in small businesses, acquire new land, and build new houses. This has all been put on hold now, affecting their socio-economic well-being and increasing their insecurity. In this liminal period, no one knows what the long-term impact of the pandemic will be. Our colleagues and newspaper articles paint diverging scenarios which range from the hope for a quick recovery of the economy to the concern that the pandemic has initiated a process of abolishing workers' rights. By highlighting gender dynamics and ethnicity, we can contend that the processes taking place in this liminal period do not only exacerbate inequalities in the labor force, thereby playing into already existing labor-related processes, but also potentially accelerate women's future exclusion from the workforce and by implication from the urban public domain.

Notes

1   www.dhakatribune.com/business/2018/03/03/womens-participation-rmg-workforce-declines/#:~:text=According%20to%20the%20survey%2C%20the,female%20and%2039.2%25%20are%20male

2   This is a co-production of activists, stakeholders, and academics. The chapter is based on in-depth ethnographic research on female garment workers and Garo beauticians between 2016 and 2018, and ongoing online communication with garment workers and local indigenous and garment workers' rights organizations.

3   The project entitled 'Migration, livelihoods and SRHR: a triple case-study of young female migrants (YFMs) in Dhaka, Bangladesh' (2016–18), was funded by the NWO/WOTRO Netherlands, and the Vrije Universiteit Amsterdam. It involved intensive collaboration with several partners and organizations in Bangladesh, including Ainoon Naher and Mirza Tasleema from the Jahangirnagar University, Meghna Guhathakurta from RIB, and partners from IPDS, BSSF, and HARC Bangladesh. Here we would in particular like to thank Runa Laila, Kathinka Sinha, Hasan Ashraf, and one other colleague who we frequently consulted for this paper and who is actively involved with labor issues in the RMG and prefers to stay anonymous.

4   www.bbc.com/news/world-asia-53420537

5   https://corona.gov.bd/?gclid=Cj0KCQjwwOz6BRCgARIsAKEG4FVBwYS0xw3yARXb_bqHytQEljpf_anc7vuJPa7gKHq9VD9-FJYcaSUaAtr8EALw_wcB)

6   While these statistics may be questionable, many months since the first outbreak the number of people dying of COVID-19 has remained remarkably low compared to several other countries.

7   www.dhakatribune.com/bangladesh/2020/08/15/health-minister-COVID-19-will-leave-bangladesh-on-its-own)

8   'The Working Poor in Bangladesh Face a "Hunger Pandemic"': www.rosalux.de/en/news/id/42864/the-working-poor-in-bangladesh-face-a-hunger-pandemic?cHash=ad4ffaedaf2a3471b5b1b15a4666afe5

9   www.bgmea.com.bd/

10   www.dw.com/en/coronavirus-economy-down-poverty-up-in-bangladesh/a-53759686

11   www.reuters.com/article/health-coronavirus-bangladesh-garments-idUSKBN29W1MG

12   www.dw.com/en/coronavirus-economy-down-poverty-up-in-bangladesh/a-53759686

13   www.newagebd.net/article/113817/156-pc-people-leave-dhaka-due-to-COVID-19-fallout-survey

[14] Although the Government of Bangladesh approved a massive bailout package of $587,925,000 for the RMG sector to pay wages, labor union activists reported the closing of factories without paying wages, massive job cuts, the firing of pregnant women, and many other actions affecting the workers' welfare. www.theguardian.com/global-development/2020/jul/09/we-are-on-our-own-bangladeshs-pregnant-garment-workers-face-the-sack See also: www.reuters.com/article/us-health-coronavirus-bangladesh-workers/bangladesh-threatens-legal-action-as-thousands-of-garment-workers-go-unpaid-idUSKCN2231N3

[15] A UN report issued towards the beginning of the pandemic positioned Bangladesh as second (4,451,000 girls) in the list of countries with the highest number of child marriages. See Share-net Bangladesh (August 24, 2020): 'Effect of COVID-19 on child marriage'. www.share-netbangladesh.org/effect-of-COVID-19-on-early-child-marriage/

References

Al-Amin, H.M., Johora, F.T. and Irish, S.R. (2020) 'Insecticide resistance status of Aedes aegypti in Bangladesh'. *Parasites Vectors*, 13(622). https://doi.org/10.1186/s13071-020-04503-6/ 10.1080/17450101.2020.1739867

Awdish, R.L.A. (2020) 'The liminal space'. *The New England Journal of Medicine*, 283(4). DOI: 10.1056/NEJMp2012147

Bal, E. (2007) *They Ask If We Eat Frogs: Garo Ethnicity in Bangladesh*. Singapore: ISEAS.

Cangià, F. (2020) 'Back to the future? Towards the post-liminal phase of COVID-19', August 8. https://blog.nccr-onthemove.ch/back-to-the-future-towards-the-post-liminal-phase-of-the-COVID-19/?lang=fr

Grabska, K. de Regt, M. and Del Franco, N. (2015) *Adolescent Girls' Migration in the Global South: Transitions into Adulthood*. Singapore: Palgrave Macmillan.

Lokot, M. and Avakyan, Y. (2020) 'Intersectionality as a lens to the COVID-19 pandemic: implications for sexual and reproductive health in development and humanitarian contexts'. *Sexual and Reproductive Health Matters*, 28(1). DOI: 10.1080/26410397.2020.1764748

Raitapuro, M. and Bal, E. (2016) ' "Talking about mobility": Garos aspiring migration and mobility in an "insecure" Bangladesh'. *South Asian History and Culture*, 7(4): 386–400.

Thomassen, B. (2009) 'The uses and meaning of liminality'. *International Political Anthropology*, 2(1): 5–28.

Van Gennep, A. (1960) *The Rites of Passage*. Chicago: University of Chicago Press.

FOURTEEN

Spatial Inequality and Colonial Palimpsest in Kuala Lumpur

Nurul Azreen Azlan

Three weeks after armed military personnel started patrolling the area and barbed wire was installed around the perimeter, an immigration raid was conducted on Menara City One and Malayan and Selangor Mansions in Kuala Lumpur, Malaysia on May 1, 2020. The irony that the raid was conducted on Labor Day was not lost, given that the three buildings were mostly populated by migrant workers living in cramped conditions. Following a spike of COVID-19 cases in early April 2020, the three buildings were put under Enforced Movement Control Order (EMCO) – a stricter version of the lockdown imposed on the rest of the country. People were prohibited from entering or leaving the buildings. Hundreds of migrants and refugees, including children, were detained in the raid, despite the Defense Minister's promise in March that punitive actions would not be taken against undocumented migrants should they come forward to get tested (Sukumaran and Jaipragas, 2020).

Malaysia performed relatively well in managing the infection rate of COVID-19 during the first wave of the pandemic. By September 2020, Malaysia had a total of 9,915 cases resulting in 128 deaths (Ministry of Health, 2020). To mitigate the impact of the pandemic, several types of lockdown were imposed depending on the number of cases and the likelihood of infection. The Movement Control Order (MCO), imposed on the whole country from March 18 to May 4, 2020 was strict: nobody was allowed to leave their homes apart from essential reasons such as getting groceries or going to the doctor. There was no mandated outdoor exercise time. For about six weeks, most people did not leave their places of residence at all.

The immigration raid was yet another pandemic episode highlighting the inherent inequality in Malaysian society. As elsewhere, the plight of the urban poor was magnified (Qamhaieh, Chapter 2; Brooks, Chapter 5; Yea, Chapter 16; Xavier, Volume 2). The lockdown meant a loss of income given the nature of their jobs that could not be done remotely, while at the same time, their expenses would have increased, given the loss of access to affordable goods and services provided by the informal markets. This was compounded by their often-cramped living conditions, making it harder for students in the household to study and follow online lessons – if it was even possible in the first place (Megat Muzafar and Kunasekaran, 2020). The ten-kilometer radius that limited people's movements, on the other hand, quickly demonstrated the uneven distribution of resources and services, an unfortunate result of uncontrolled and sprawling development.

While the relatively low number of infections in Malaysia may point towards successful mitigation measures by the state, the aforementioned incident also revealed the racist and classist assumptions, further magnified by the vitriol found online against migrants and refugees. The intersection of medical practices and armed forces, marginalized communities and overcrowding, sanitation and the policing of space, are reminiscent of colonial methods of ordering space – as observed by Franz Fanon in *The Wretched of the Earth* (1963: 37) – and society.

Sanitation and the colonial ordering of space

Owing its prosperity to tin mining, Kuala Lumpur grew from a sparsely populated settlement into a city in the 1850s. By the time the British moved their base from Klang to Kuala Lumpur, there were already some patterns of spatial segregation according to ethnicity and belief, which fit rather well with British policy (King, 2008). Europeans in general constituted a minority in Malayan towns, with many of them taking up residence in the plantations or in the Straits Settlements (Lees, 2011: 50). Their presence in town would be marked by a more stringent form of segregation, since the colonials sought to minimize contact and conflict with the Others, thus providing the Europeans with a high degree of comfort (Dick and Rimmer, 1998: 2308). Race was, after all, a defining feature of colonial planning (King, 1977). It was this racialized structure that the national elites ended up inheriting after independence, along with a pluralist worldview (Goh, 2008: 234).

This hierarchy and segregation were naturally extended to the provision of colonial medical practices and sanitation. Colonial medical practices would prioritize the Europeans first, then the migrant labor force, and finally the native population if their situation might prove threatening to the well-being of the Europeans (Manderson, 1999). Physical separation of races became a sanitation device in the colony – incidentally, the term segregation to denote separation of races also arose around the same time as the term town planning (Home, 2014: 80).

Housing and sanitation for the natives were also typically underfunded, and this, together with the chronic unsanitary conditions of native housing, was justified using colonial discourse of Otherness – that the natives were incapable of maintaining a sanitary environment (Chang et al, 2013: 57). This Otherness would muddle otherwise well-meaning municipal interventions with prejudices based on race, culture, color, and class (King, 1977).

Thus, the limited resources would be disproportionately invested to further improve the environs and sanitation of the already high-quality districts where Europeans resided. Meanwhile, the poorest could rent a room or cubicle for their whole family in the tenements, sharing common facilities such as kitchen and toilets with other families (Chang et al, 2013: 57).

The use of colonial medical practices and sanitation as an apparatus of control and discipline is well-documented (Fanon, 1965; Lees, 2011). As Fanon (1965) observed in Algeria, a visit to the doctor would be followed by a visit by the army since the doctor would take note of the patient's information together with those accompanying them. In Malaya, the British would use Sanitary Boards to indirectly control populations, while relying on the police force for a more direct form of discipline (Lees, 2011). Sanitation and governance were tightly linked in practice and in the minds of colonial officials (Lees, 2011: 55). It is no coincidence that the first urban authority set up during the colonial administration of Kuala Lumpur was the Sanitary Board in 1890, the precursor of the present-day City Hall (Lepawsky and Jubilado, 2014: 28).

Thus, the emergence of planning in the colony was very much colored by segregation as an acceptable planning tool, since segregation by race was seen as a crucial sanitation measure. This assumption was propagated by racist colonial discourse that denoted the inability of the indigenous and migrant labor force to maintain a sanitary environment was due to their inherent cultural flaws.

Inequality in the city

Malayan and Selangor Mansions are areas with large concentrations of migrants and are situated in the Malay/Indian Muslim quarter of old Kuala Lumpur, within the vicinity of the historic core. Built in the early post-independence years, these blocks of flats saw their glory days in the 1960s (Soo,

2020). Selangor Mansion used to be home to shoemaking and textile pioneers in the city, and renowned painter Chia You Chian called it home for 45 years (Soo, 2020). According to the Defense Minister, at the time of the EMCO, there were 6,000 residents living in 365 residential and commercial units. That would mean that an average of 16 people were living in a two-bedroom flat.

Similarly, Kampong Baru, a Malay urban village within walking distance of the Mansions also ended up with an EMCO. Kampong Baru was set up as a Malay Reserve by the British administrators in 1900, to balance the presence of the Chinese in Kuala Lumpur (King, 2008). Comprising mostly of Malay kampong houses, the urban form of Kampong Baru is more suburban in comparison with the tight urban fabric around the Selangor and Malayan Mansions. Even though the urban form of Kampong Baru is vastly different from the area around the Mansions, it still recorded a high number of cases (110) as of May 6 (Ministry of Health, 2020). However, both areas are strategically situated within the city center, making them very attractive to migrant workers in the service sector around the city. Just as an average of 16 people were cramped into the two-bedroom flats in the Mansions, the authorities discovered that 70 people were living in a house in Kampong Baru after it caught fire. In cases such as this, homeowners no longer lived there and could charge up to RM15,000 (approximately $3,600) rent a month given its premium location, thus laying down the conditions for overcrowding.

The central parts of Malaysian cities, especially Kuala Lumpur, are unaffordable. A person living in central Kuala Lumpur is either wealthy enough to afford the astronomical rent, and probably identifies as an expatriate – or they are poor and most likely a dark-skinned migrant worker, and the only way to afford their accommodation is to live in cramped conditions. It would be very difficult for them to maintain a safe physical distance from each other, given the overcrowded situation. Hence, it came as no surprise when there was a spike of cases in these areas known to host migrant workers.

The Selayang Wholesale Market, situated just outside the city, was also shut down due to the EMCO and subsequently raided. Supposedly run by Rohingyan gangsters, the EMCO invited some unsavory comments on social media about the Rohingyans, signifying a change of heart from the welcoming stance taken by the public when trouble first started brewing in Myanmar. A lot of the comments focused on the purportedly unsanitary habits of the Rohingyans, such as spitting betel leaf juice everywhere, and also a general untrustworthiness. Refugees are not allowed to work in Malaysia, which makes supporting themselves through legal means very difficult. However, some have observed that lighter-skinned refugees such as those from Syria and Bosnia in the 1990s were treated with more warmth. Confronted with this contradiction, the usual excuse is these lighter-skinned refugees are better behaved than their dark-skinned brethren.

Similar vitriol was also hurled at the residents of the Mansions. They were accused of being unsanitary and leeching off public money. The Defense Minister even said that the government would not be providing food, encouraging the respective embassies to provide for their citizens.

Blanket enforcement of orders was also put in place, without any nuance apart from one of class. For example, all foreigners were banned from entering religious spaces and wholesale markets. Refugees entering wholesale markets had to be accompanied by a Malaysian. The immigration sweeps also resulted in the detainment of those whose tourist visa had lapsed during the MCO – one such person from India contracted COVID-19 in the detention center and lost their life. The Benteng Cluster for example, refers to 403 cases in a detention center caused by cramped conditions. The Defense Minister initially announced that citizens of countries with more than 150,000 cases would not be allowed to enter Malaysia, however, the ban was relaxed for expatriates and professional visit pass-holders after protests by employers. At the same time, the work permit of Mohamad Rayhan Kabir, a Bangladeshi, was revoked, and he was then deported – for criticizing the government over their handling of undocumented migrants in a documentary produced by Al-Jazeera.

The city as a colonial palimpsest

These incidents triggered by the COVID-19 lockdown echo colonial attitudes. The immigration raids on the Mansions and the Selayang Wholesale Market were where the colonial apparatus of public health and policing converged, and the pandemic provided a public health excuse to conduct an immigration sweep. However, no discernible actions were taken against those who would have been part of the supply chain of migrant workers, all the impact was borne by the migrant workers themselves. The poor housing condition in the tenements evokes the housing provided to the poorest of the poor during colonial times. This is also applicable to the cramped conditions in detention centers that have caused massive spikes of infection (see also Yea, Chapter 16). On October 6, 2020, half of the cases announced at the COVID-19 daily press conference came from a prison in Kedah, a state in the northern part of peninsula Malaysia. And yet, the situation was still deemed under control, simply because they were contained and had no contact with society at large.

As Dick and Rimmer (1998: 2317) astutely observed, the attitudes of the middle class in Southeast Asia towards the urban mass are not that different from those of colonial Europeans towards the indigenous subjects. Public space was to be avoided since it might mean contact with the Other, who is potentially dangerous and would cause discomfort. The vitriol hurled at the migrant workers over their living conditions evoke the colonial discourse of Otherness, justifying the cramped conditions and poor sanitation as a result of cultural differences – the role of employers and employment agents who are most likely responsible for the provision of housing and at times even cause the otherwise legal migrant workers to become undocumented is rarely discussed (Sukumaran and Jaipragas, 2020).

The inequality laid bare by the pandemic has demonstrated that there is a tendency to imitate colonial attitudes, even 63 years after Malaya became independent from the British. The fact that Kuala Lumpur's City Hall originated from the British Sanitary Board makes one question the underlying ethos and assumptions they currently have about governing the city, given the colonial practice of racial segregation as an acceptable measure of sanitation. The pandemic has shown that there is an urgent need to reflect upon our colonial heritage, and to decolonize urban planning in Malaysia.

References

Chang, J.H., Peckham, R. and Pomfret, D.M. (2013) ' "Tropicalizing" planning: sanitation, housing, and technologies of improvement in colonial Singapore'. *Imperial Contagions: Medicine, Hygiene, and Cultures of Planning in Asia*, 37.

Dick, H.W. and Rimmer, P.J. (1998) 'Beyond the third world city: the new urban geography of South-east Asia'. *Urban Studies*, 35(12): 2303–21.

Fanon, F. (1963) *The Wretched of the Earth*. Translated by C. Farrington. New York: Grove Press.

Fanon, F. (1965) *A Dying Colonialism*. New York: Grove Press.

Goh, D.P.S. (2008) 'From colonial pluralism to postcolonial multiculturalism: race, state formation and the question of cultural diversity in Malaysia and Singapore'. *Sociology Compass*, 2(1): 232–52.

Home, R. (2014) 'Legal histories of planning and colonialism', in S. Parnell and S. Oldfield (eds) *The Routledge Handbook on Cities of the Global South*. New York: Routledge, p 75.

King, A. (1977) 'Exporting "planning": the colonial and neo-colonial experience'. *Urbanism Past & Present*, 5: 12–22.

King, R. (2008) *Kuala Lumpur and Putrajaya Negotiating Urban Space in Malaysia*. Asian Studies Association of Australia in association with University of Hawaii Press.

Lees, L. (2011) 'Discipline and delegation: colonial governance in Malayan towns, 1880–1930'. *Urban History*, 38(1): 48–64.

Lepawsky, J. and Jubilado, R.C. (2014) 'Globalising Kuala Lumpur and rationalising the street: hawkers and the aporias of urban renewal along Petaling Street and Jalan Masjid India', in Y.S. Guan (ed) *The Other Kuala Lumpur: Living in the Shadows of a Globalising Southeast Asian City*. New York: Routledge, pp 22–40.

Manderson, L. (1999) 'Public health developments in colonial Malaya: colonialism and the politics of prevention'. *American Journal of Public Health*, 89(1): 102–07.

Megat Muzafar, P.M. and Kunasekaran, T. (2020) 'The impact of Covid-19 on the urban poor: three major threats – money, food and living conditions'. Kuala Lumpur: Khazanah Research Institute.

Ministry of Health (2020) 'Jumlah Pecahan Kes Mengikut Daerah, Zon dan Presint', Situasi Terkini 07 Mei 2020. Retrieved from: http://covid-19.moh.gov.my/terkini/052020/situasi-terkini-07-mei-2020

Soo, W.J. (2020) 'Covid-19: Selangor Mansion's history a far cry from its rundown present'. *Malay Mail*. Retrieved from: www.malaymail.com

Sukumaran, T. and Jaipragas, B. (2020) 'Coronavirus: hundreds arrested as Malaysia cracks down on migrants in Covid-19 red zones'. *South China Morning Post*. Retrieved from: www.scmp.com

FIFTEEN

The COVID-19 Pandemic and the Travails of Rohingya Refugees in the Largest Bangladeshi Refugee Camp

Diotima Chattoraj, AKM Ahsan Ullah, and

Mallik Akram Hossain

Introduction

COVID-19 has been labeled a 'pandemic', which turned out to be one of the most terrifying diseases causing an impending crisis the world has not witnessed in the recent era (Chattoraj, 2021). Before the development of successful vaccines, the World Health Organization's (WHO) recommendations such as quarantining, wearing masks, self-isolating, maintaining social distance, and lockdown were the only measures available to combat COVID-19 (Ullah et al, 2021). However, these are not always feasible for all communities (see Lemanski and de Groot, Chapter Ten); for the refugees living in small and overcrowded tiny shacks that are found in refugee camps, a major challenge lies in maintaining social distance and lockdown measures. Rohingya refugees in Bangladesh, who were forced out of the Northern Rakhine State of Myanmar in the face of brutal persecution, rapes, and killings are no exception (Ullah and Chattoraj, 2018).

There are an estimated 1.2 million Rohingya refugees staying in 34 camps (Bhuyian, 2021) outside Cox's Bazar, a district of southeast Bangladesh (Ullah and Chattoraj, 2021). They face a heightened risk of COVID-19 owing to poor, cramped conditions and densely populated camps. They lack access to adequate health care, shelter, water, and sanitation, which pose major challenges in their efforts to protect themselves from the virus. Therefore, the main objective of this chapter is to provide details about these challenges, and the experiences of the Rohingyas in these refugee camps due to the sudden emergence of the pandemic.

During the initial phases of the outbreak, health experts from the United Nations High Commissioner for Refugees (UNHCR) and International Organization for Migration (IOM) warned that if the virus reached the world's largest refugee camp, it would spread like wildfire and Bangladesh might become devastated by COVID-19 due to the arrangements of camp settlements. The population density in the Rohingya camp is more than 100,000 people per square mile and sanitation options are scarce. Groceries, kiosks, health centers, and schools are all located within the camps, making congestion worse (Ullah et al, 2020). These camps are overcrowded as many families have more than ten members living in one room. Severely substandard health care and inadequate access to proper sanitation have made them incredibly vulnerable to this virus.

The context

The virus first hit the Rohingya camp in Bangladesh in March 2020. By April, 2021, around 507 Rohingyas had tested positive, eleven of whom had died (Sakib, 2021). While this number is low, one must realize the grave situation that these camps are facing. Rohingya refugee camps are located outside the town of Cox's Bazaar and are clearly demarcated – fenced – defining a distinction between the refugees on the inside and the locals on the outside. Having been established to prevent the contamination of Bangladesh and its citizens by the Rohingya refugees, it is important to the government to establish and maintain this distinction between the inside and the outside. In practice, the camps allow exchange of goods, ideas, and movement of people in and out of the camp. Despite these transgressions of the limits of the camp, the perimeter remains an important defining characteristic and shapes the lives of those who remain inside. Living inside a refugee camp – however invisible the line between the camp and its surroundings, and despite ongoing contact between the inside and the outside – marks one's life and defines one's position: a position that is simultaneously excluded from and included into host society, excluded spatially and legally while simultaneously being defined and contained by the surrounding society (Turner, 2015).

Hence, refugees and the host society are related. The new COVID-19 slogan 'Stay Home, Stay Safe' (Ullah et al, 2021) is a double-edged sword for the refugees as most of them are engaged in daily labors outside the camps. Also, maintaining social distance is an impossible task where families share toilets and handwashing facilities. Due to limited mobility and transport opportunities, they are also deprived of accessing hospitals in times of need (Ullah et al, 2020). This leads their health status to remain extremely fragile.

Therefore, the national government and its partners need to look after these refugees. If refugees are left in this precarious condition, it could lead to the increased risk of locals contracting COVID-19 as they come in direct contact with them.

Methodology

For this study, we depended mostly on an 'Internet search' (Chattoraj, 2017) including a wide range of online reports, documents, and newspaper articles. Informal interviews were conducted remotely via telephone with 57 Rohingya refugees, aged between 18 and 55 years, residing in the Kutupalong camp in Bangladesh. We were in touch with one of the research groups in Chittagong, Bangladesh and through them, we obtained the contacts of our respondents. Because the Chittagong research group was working closely with the Rohingyas in the camps, we did not face many problems in establishing a rapport and building up trust with them. Being Bengali native speakers, language did not create any issues. All the interviews were conducted in Bengali and then translated into English. In addition to these refugees, a number of volunteers, health workers, and representatives of local and international organizations were also interviewed.

This pandemic created new challenges in collecting data, as we were not allowed to roam freely and talk with whoever we wanted to speak with. We needed special permission from Security to enter the camps, which was not granted, so we were not allowed to enter, and thus had to solely depend on our phone interviews with the refugees. This can also be considered as a limitation of this study.

Rohingya camps and COVID-19: the challenges

With the current COVID-19 pandemic affecting innumerable livelihoods and plunging the global economy into a recession, questions have arisen as to the well-being of the Rohingyas who are languishing in overcrowded refugee camps. Their camps comprise an area of about 40,000 people per square kilometer (103,600 per square mile) where refugees live in tiny shacks side by side (Ullah et al, 2020). Each of these shacks is barely ten square meters (107 square feet). Thus, these jam-packed camps have made their lives incredibly vulnerable to this virus.

'We witnessed and experienced heart wrenching and inhuman violence, and brutalities (in the form of killings, lynching, rapes, beatings) perpetrated on us and our families in Rakhine. Those memories haunt us all the time. Was it not enough that this COVID-19 has to haunt us now? How can we survive?'

This was one of the most common sentiments that we heard from the Rohingyas during our interviews. They had already seen quite a lot, but it seems that was not enough. Most of them were still suffering from past traumas. With COVID-19, now they have lost all hope of surviving.

Challenges involving mobility

To stem the COVID-19 pandemic, on March 26, 2020, the entire Cox's Bazar district, including the camps, began their lockdowns for an indefinite period (Ullah et al, 2020). As one respondent noted: "Lockdown has become a nightmare. We are dependent on the inflow of supplies, medical services and materials from outside, and also many among us routinely go out for work." Only emergency health services and distribution of foods are allowed in the camps and the refugees are banned from roaming about unnecessarily. Another respondent said, "These days, we had to wait for more than four hours in the queue to get food and materials. […] we had to wait until we were called." Vehicles moving into the camps for emergency reasons are only allowed with proper permissions from higher authorities (Ullah et al, 2020). Schools, learning centers, and social places have been shut over fears of the virus. COVID-19 has changed everything in the camp, said the respondents in a frightened tone: "The mosques are empty; children, instead of playing in the streets, are now confined to their huts and the bustling markets are quiet. Families are forced to ration food and spend all day together in cramped spaces."

Health challenges

The cramped and overcrowded camps are generally dangerous and unsanitary as aid agencies struggle to keep pace with the needs of the ever-growing Rohingya (Ullah and Chattoraj, 2021). As their number grows, their living space becomes more congested in the camps, which in turn increases their health risks. About 85 percent of the Rohingya still have no access to latrines, exposing them to increased risk of communicable diseases (Ullah and Chattoraj, 2021). "So you see, there is not enough running water for every one of us to wash our hands."

Rohingyas suffer from several diseases like TB, malaria, malnutrition, measles, diphtheria, diarrhea, dysentery, and so on (Ullah and Chattoraj, 2021). At least 60 percent of water wells in the camps are contaminated with fecal matter from latrines that have been dug too close to drinking sources, leading to these diseases.

The UN, together with partner organizations, has constructed isolation and treatment centers inside the camps. They have started promoting hygiene activities, training health care workers, and ensuring social distancing across the camps. Self-isolation and social distancing have become new normals. However, the large crowds of refugees are not interested in paying attention to the social distancing guidelines (Anik, 2020). Nor are they keen to wear face masks, which have become one of the daily essentials in today's world.

The Bangladesh Government's new directive protects 'critical' services including health, nutrition, water, food, gas, hygiene, sanitation, waste treatment, identification of new arrivals, and 'ensuring quarantine'. However, internet restrictions have facilitated the spread of misinformation, deterring refugees from seeking urgent medical care in times of COVID-19. In addition, a reduction in the number of aid workers in the camps is causing another threat to refugees because this has halted other vaccination programs, such as against measles and rubella. While the national government has partnered with the COVAX Facility to allocate 5% of its COVID-19 vaccines for refugees, it is yet unclear when Rohingya camps will receive doses (IRC, 2021).

The Rohingyas have expressed serious concerns about the rainy season causing a deterioration in camp roads, paths, and stair networks thereby impacting access to necessary services and amplifying a multitude of protection issues such as physical and sexual abuse. Annual monsoon preparations in the camps were made more challenging with the risks posed by COVID-19. Though the number of cases in the camps are low, there is evidence of large-scale spread of the disease among them (Anik, 2020). Instead of going to the testing centers, several refugees are flocking to pharmacies, seeking treatment for cough or fever – primary symptoms of the deadly virus. Also, the poor quality of medication and equipment used in treatment centers are also part of the reasons refugees are against getting tested (Anik, 2020).

Economic challenges

Pre-COVID-19 days saw some of the refugees having set up several stalls on roadsides throughout the camps. On the one hand, girls were sent to work as maids for the locals, or in the local garment industry (Ullah and Chattoraj, 2021). On the other hand, boys used to work in tea stalls or would provide manual labor for construction sites and road crews (Ullah and Chattoraj, 2021). The lockdown has restricted their movements. Because of this, they are suffering economically. They are scared, tense and hapless and are worried about their uncertain future, as summarized by one respondent: "If we cannot go out, we cannot work and if we cannot work, who will give us money? We will die of hunger!"

Conclusion

Despite attempts to separate refugees from the locals, Darling (2017: 181) argues that 'the continuing attraction of the town/city for the refugees is clear, as the city can represent a site of independence and safety not necessarily found in camps'. Following Darling (2017), we can observe that several studies have explored the livelihood opportunities of refugees, highlighting both the integration of individuals into an informal economy of casual labor and the continued vulnerability of such individuals to abuse, arrest, and harassment. This tension, as portrayed by Darling (2017), between the prospects of temporary safety and opportunity, and the risks of exploitation and marginalization is an often-repeated one in explorations of urban refugee experiences, evident in the works of Jacobsen (2006), Crawley et al (2019), Chattoraj (2018), Chattoraj and Gerharz (2019), and several others.

In pre-COVID-19 days, they were often referred to as Barmaiya by the locals which means 'from Burma' in an offensive manner. Thus, they were socially excluded from locals because of their 'refugee' status. Their experiences of social exclusion and the process of 'othering' kept on increasing due to the pandemic. They became more isolated from locals as they were no longer allowed to intermingle with the outsiders.

Because of the uncertainties prevailing in the camps, several young refugees, desperate with their situation, used to risk their lives and seek out illegal and dangerous ways to get themselves to third countries (Ullah and Chattoraj, 2021). Due to COVID-19 they are left with no other choice other than to stay in the camps and suffer economically and socially. The locals in Cox's Bazar demand the repatriation of the refugees to Myanmar. To them, 'the Rohingya pose a threat to the locals' as they are stealing jobs from the locals. In this chapter, we have shown the existence of urban inequities among the locals and the Rohingyas in the age of COVID-19. The pandemic exacerbates the gap between the two protagonists as the Rohingyas remain in complete isolation from the rest of the country.

References

Anik, S.S.B. (2020) 'Covid-19 in Rohingya Refugee Camps'. *Dhaka Tribune*, August 24. Retrieved from: www.dhakatribune.com/bangladesh/rohingya-crisis/2020/08/24/covid-19-in-rohingya-refugee-camps

Bhuyian, H.K. (2021) 'Bangladesh successful in protecting Rohingyas from Covid-19'. *Dhaka Tribune*, March 9. Retrieved from: www.dhakatribune.com/health/coronavir us/2021/03/09/bangladesh-s-success-in-protecting-rohingyas-from-covid-19

Chattoraj, D. (2017) *Ambivalent attachments: shifting notions of home among displaced Sri Lankan Tamils*. Doctoral dissertation, Ruhr-Universität Bochum.

Chattoraj, D. (2018) 'Narratives of Sri Lankan displaced Tamils living in welfare centers in Jaffna, Sri Lanka'. *Journal of Maritime Studies and National Integration*, 2(2): 67–74.

Chattoraj, D. (2021) 'The grateful migrants: Indians and Bangladeshis in Singapore in times of Covid-19'. *South East Asia: A Multidisciplinary Journal*, 20(2): 44–62.

Chattoraj, D. and Gerharz, E. (2019) 'Strangers at home: narratives of northern Muslim returnees in post-war Sri Lanka'. *Sri Lanka Journal of Social Sciences*, 42(2): 113–26.

Crawley, H., Drinkwater, S. and Kausar, R. (2019) 'Attitudes towards asylum seekers: understanding differences between rural and urban areas'. *Journal of Rural Studies*, 71: 104–13.

Darling, J. (2017) 'Forced migration and the city: irregularity, informality, and the politics of presence'. *Progress in Human Geography*, 41(2): 178–98.

International Rescue Committee (IRC) (2021) 'As Covid-19 vaccines begin reaching conflict and crisis settings, [...]'. April 27. Retrieved from: www.rescue-uk.org/press-release/covid-19-vaccines-begin-reaching-conflict-and-crisis-settings-new-study-highlights

Jacobsen, K. (2006) 'Refugees and asylum seekers in urban areas: a livelihoods perspective'. *Journal of Refugee Studies*, 19(3): 273–86.

Sakib, S.M.N. (2021) 'Covid-19 kills 11 Rohingya refugees in Bangladesh camps'. Anadolu Agency (AA), April 21. Retrieved from: www.aa.com.tr/en/asia-pacific/covid-19-kills-11-rohingya-refugees-in-bangladesh-camps/2215278

Turner, S. (2015) 'What is a refugee camp? Explorations of the limits and effects of the camp'. *Journal of Refugee Studies*, 29(2).

Ullah, A.K.M.A. and Chattoraj, D. (2018) 'Roots of discrimination against Rohingya minorities: society, ethnicity and international relations'. *Intellectual Discourse*, 26(2): 541–65.

Ullah, A.K.M.A. and Chattoraj, D. (2021) 'Rohingya children in Bangladesh: questioning the past and imagining the future', in K. Alijunied (ed) *Routledge Handbook of Islam in Southeast Asia*. New York: Routledge.

Ullah, A.K.M.A., Hossain, M.A. and Chattoraj, D. (2020) 'Covid-19 and Rohingya refugee camps in Bangladesh'. *Intellectual Discourse*, 28(2): 793–806.

Ullah, A.K.M.A., Nawaz, F. and Chattoraj, D. (2021) 'Locked under lockdown: the COVID-19 pandemic and the migrant population'. *Social Sciences & Humanities Open*, 3(1): 100126.

SIXTEEN

Singapore's Pandemic Governance and Deepening Marginalization of Migrant Workmen

Sallie Yea

Introduction

In the early stages of the COVID-19 pandemic in February 2020, Singapore appeared to have control over the spread of the virus among the general population. This changed quickly, however, in late March 2020, when several new clusters of infection emerged, and the number of cases soared. By early April, Singapore had one of the highest rates of infection per capita of anywhere in the world. Beneath this startling statistic is a complex picture of migrant worker infection clusters connected to a structural and institutional history of socio-spatial exclusion and economic marginalization (see also Azlan, Chapter Fourteen). It is this structural regime that arguably helped produce a situation by April 2020, where over 90 percent of Singapore's infections and all major infection clusters were located among the thousands of transient migrant workmen, predominantly from South Asia, working in the city state.

The chapter examines the governance of migrants through urban space in 'pandemic times'. Migrant workers represent a group with heightened vulnerability to infection due to their precarious working and living conditions. I argue that this vulnerability, as well as the early responses to the pandemic, which largely excluded migrant workers, has produced intense pandemic governance of migrant workers vis-à-vis the citizen/permanent resident population. I argue that these two aspects of migrant worker precarity are mutually reinforcing; vulnerability to infection is shaped by a pre-existing political economy of governance that contains and marginalizes migrant workmen, with responses to this heightened vulnerability reinforcing and exacerbating these very same processes of containment and marginalization. In the chapter I draw out how these processes are simultaneously spatialized and racialized and suggest they may help perpetuate a divisive post-pandemic urban governance of migrants.

The chapter first briefly reviews the racial/migrant context of Singapore and policies aimed at the spatialization of difference. I then examine the living and working conditions of these migrant workmen in Singapore to help explain the prevalence of COVID-19 infections among this sub-population. In this part of the chapter I pay particular attention to the spatialization of migrant workmen's working and living conditions and the causality of these situations in the current infection trends. The third part of the chapter examines the measures to contain the spread of COVID-19 and reduce infection rates in the city state that were introduced in the second quarter of 2020. In this part of the chapter I connect the responses to early phases of the pandemic with broader, pre-existing urban/migrant governance measures.

The spatialization of racial differentiation in Singapore's migrant worker governance

Migrant workers comprise approximately one third of Singapore's total population at any given time (Ministry of

Manpower, 2019), with migrant workmen engaged in two-year contracts in the construction, shipyard, and landscaping sectors comprising approximately 400,000 of these transient workers. The majority of these men are nationals of Bangladesh, India (especially Tamil Nadu), and the People's Republic of China respectively. While these men play a vital role in underpinning Singapore's competitiveness in key sectors of the economy, they are generally regarded with distain by the general public and are stereotyped as threatening, dirty, and dangerous (Goh, 2019). This perception plays an important causative role in guiding state policies governing migrant worker incorporation in Singapore and in regulating (or not adequately regulating) their working and living conditions.

Singapore has a complex racial mosaic comprising a citizenry that is predominantly ethnic Chinese, with Indian and Malay minorities. Foreign residents in Singapore include both transient migrant workers and permanent residents. Transient migrant workers on short-term contracts (normally two years) are incorporated through a national quota system in which selected source countries for specific Work Permit Holder (WPH) roles, such as construction worker or domestic helper, are allowed a specific number of visa entrants. In addition to the predominantly South Asian and Chinese construction, shipyard and landscaping visas, the Philippines, Indonesia, Sri Lanka, Bangladesh, and India also have visa quotas for paid domestic work. A range of other nationalities are also represented in the hospitality and service sector. The vast numbers of South Asian unskilled migrant workmen are viewed by both the Singapore government and the general public as a necessary evil (Velayutham, 2009). Various incidents have reinforced this perception. In recent times the so-called Little India 'Riot' in December 2013 was the most infamous of these. This incident saw Tamil migrant workers set fire to vehicles and vandalize shopfronts and emergency vehicles after a Tamil worker was run over by a bus and killed. While non-government organizations pushed for recognizing the key role played by underlying migrant worker precarity and exploitation in explaining the riot, government discourse centered on the unmediated violence of a 'mob' (Kaur et al, 2016).

One of the main consequences of the emerging public anxieties around migrant workmen has been the drive to spatially and socially separate this group from the general population. One such incident occurred when neighboring residents protested at the planned conversion of a disused school in the upperclass neighborhood of Serangoon Gardens into a dormitory for migrant workmen in 2008. The residents' collective concerns were articulated as a fall in the value of their properties and the potential danger such a dormitory would pose to residents' safety. To appease the residents, the government constructed a fence around the dormitory and included recreational facilities on-site, thereby discouraging worker-residents from spilling out into neighboring parks and public spaces.

As with the response to the Serangoon Gardens dispute, the Singapore government, acting primarily through Singapore's Urban Redevelopment Authority (URA), Ministry of Manpower (MOM), and a number of other government agencies, has implemented a migrant workmen governance regime that has resulted in the socio-spatial regulation and de facto segregation of workmen (Ye, 2016). Foremost among these interventions has been the governance of migrant workman housing through the introduction of purpose-built dormitories (PBDs), which can contain upwards of several thousand men each. These PBDs are self-contained with all amenities to service the residents' daily needs located within the dormitory site itself. This includes canteens, a centralized kitchen and dining hall, laundry, sickbay and chemist, barber's shop, outdoor games courts and recreation/socializing areas, minimart, fitness center and gymnasium, open field, and indoor recreation facilities such as a TV lounge. There are 13 PBDs in Singapore that are governed by the Building and Construction Authority (BCA), whose management is contracted out to private operators (BCA, nd). Without exception, these PBDs are constructed in outlying areas of Singapore where there are few other residential dwellings nearby.

Companies employing migrant workmen are not yet formally required to accommodate their workers in these PBDs. However, other sites commonly housing these workers – such as in shipping containers on or near construction sites, in HDB (high-density blocks) flats, and in rooms above shopfronts – are subject to increasing restrictions on their use and, in the case of shopfronts, repurposing through urban redevelopment aimed at gentrification. The decline in alternative accommodation that is more 'embedded' in the everyday fabric of Singapore and where encounters with local residents more likely have led to an expansion in the number of occupants in PBD and their promotion by the government as the most appropriate accommodation for workers. In addition to the promotion of one specific housing option, various agents of the government (police in particular) undertake regular 'urban cleansing' operations in publics spaces where migrant workers' presence is deemed undesirable. Publics parks, shopping malls, and communal areas of HDBs are often targeted in these efforts (Transient Workers Count Too (TWC2), 2012). In short, in Singapore the government has instituted a policy of socio-spatial separation of migrant workmen from the general population. This policy is based both on entrenched racism and a perception that male migrant Others are dangerous and unruly.

Migrant precarity and the production of pandemic 'hotspots'

Several studies have documented the precarity of transient migrant workers in Singapore, including practices such as wage theft, disciplining and punishing workers, and the imposition of fraudulent contracts and condition papers (Humanitarian Organisation for Migrant Economies (HOME and TWC2), 2010; Yea and Chok, 2018). Others have identified the particular health vulnerabilities migrant workers suffer, including heightened exposure to injury (Chok, 2014) and infection (Yea, 2017). Arguably, migrant workmen's substandard living and working conditions have predisposed them to heightened vulnerability to COVID-19 inflection. Living conditions that have contributed to this heightened vulnerability include cramped, overcrowded, and unhygienic accommodation, crowded work and transport spaces, and poor-quality food, among others (Dutta, 2018). Whether workers live in PBDs or other forms of housing, overcrowding and lack of hygiene are ongoing problems.

In early March 2020 community transmission of COVID-19 was already occurring in Singapore, and interventions were swiftly introduced by Singapore's Ministry of Health. These included the issuing of face masks to all citizens and residents, though this excluded migrant workmen. Social distancing was introduced in public eating venues, and offices and other workplaces were asked to stagger employee attendance so as to make social distancing requirements possible. Personal hygiene was also subject to increasing regulation, including frequent handwashing and the use of hand sanitizers. A partial lockdown was also implemented in what the government labeled a 'circuit breaker' to reduce community transmission.

As the earlier responses suggest, a racialized and nationalized divide between those who were and were not included under these measures began to emerge. The availability of masks, the ability to maintain basic hygiene in unhygienic living and working quarters, the ability to stagger work, and social distancing practices at both the workplace and in places of residence were all denied to migrant workmen in these initial responses. Migrant workmen were still expected to work and were ferried to and from their workplaces to their housing in crowded conditions, often shoulder to shoulder on the backs of lorries (personal communication, Debbie Fordyce, TWC2, April 14, 2020). In their workplaces, they came into close contact with other workers from different companies and residential arrangements, returning to their own dormitories where they were often sharing the same room with upwards of 20 other men.

It was only when clusters of COVID-19 infection began to emerge among migrant workmen in these situations that new interventions targeted specifically at this sub-population were introduced. Opondo and Shapino (2020) argue that during the COVID-19 pandemic bodies have been marked in particular ways; essential and non-essential, with and without pre-existing conditions, and located in, 'precarious zones of abandonment, congestion and containment'. The emerging biopolitical marking of migrant workmen as a risk group, albeit one arguably created by a combination of the shortcomings of early interventions and long-standing migrant worker precarity, portended new types of interventions that arguably marked these migrants as in need of containment. These included strict isolation of workmen in their dormitory rooms and the removal of some non-infected workmen to floating accommodation in Singapore's harbor. In sum, at the core of the Singapore government's circuit breaker response was the containment and confinement of migrant workmen. Arguably, such responses further embedded pre-existing policies that divided this group from the general population and gave further impetus and legitimacy to such measures.

Conclusion

In this chapter I have taken the view in line with many other chapters in this series that the risk of COVID-19 infection is, in part, an outcome of pre-existing disadvantage and marginalization. For migrant workmen this has meant both the inability to contest employment situations that may further heighten this risk and their exclusion from interventions that could enhance their protection against infection. This inequitable distribution of risk has been discussed in relation to other diseases, such as tuberculosis. Craig (2007) suggests that the discourses of risk in public health responses circulate along particular gendered and racial/ethnic lines. Prevention and care both circulate through these discourses, which come to influence interventions. I have also suggested in the chapter that migrants have been construed in pandemic discourses in Singapore as a threat to be contained (a risk *to* society), rather than COVID-19 being construed as a threat to migrant workers' health (a risk *for* migrant workmen). This discursive rendering lay behind the differential health interventions targeting citizens and permanent residents vis-à-vis migrant workmen.

In Singapore, as elsewhere, COVID-19 governance is profoundly spatial; aimed at population containment, isolation, removal, and (im)mobility. In cities, where the concentration of population is often greatest, these spatialities are intensely expressed. In this chapter I have made a two-fold argument about the interstices between urban pandemic governance, race, and transient migrants in Singapore. First, I have suggested that migrant workmen experience heightened vulnerability to COVID-19 infection due to pre-existing living and working conditions, and that this vulnerability is reproduced and heightened during the immediate, short-term pandemic governance. Second, I have suggested that, in the longer term, management of pandemic 'risk' that identifies migrant workmen as particularly risky bodies enables the pursuit of policies that deepen the already emerging socio-spatial divide between migrant workmen and the general population. Separating analysis of the immediacy of pandemic infection control from the longer-term state goal of building post-pandemic resilience allows us to identify how government responses are both discrete and compounding. Other implications of divisive pandemic governance in Singapore are noteworthy and are worthy of further examination. In both their initial vulnerability and in government responses to COVID-19, migrant workmen's positions of disposability have been intensely deepened.

References

BCA (nd) www1.bca.gov.sg/buildsg/manpower/foreign-worker-dormitories

Chok, S. (2014) 'Risky business: death and injury on Singapore's construction sites'. Singapore: Health Serve. Retrieved from: www.researchgate.net/publication/312913824_Risky_Business_Death_Injury_on_Singapore's_Construction_Sites_Examining_Worksite_UnSafety_Through_Conversations_with_Migrant_Construction_Workers

Craig, G.M. (2007) 'Nation, "migration" and tuberculosis'. *Social Theory and Health*, 5: 267–84.

Dutta, M.J. (2018) 'Negotiating health on dirty jobs: culture-centred constructions of health among migrant construction workers in Singapore', in Y. Mao and R. Ahmed (eds) *Culture, Migration and Health Communication in a Global Context*. New York: Routledge, pp 1–15.

Goh, D.P.S. (2019) 'Superdiversity and the biopolitics of migrant worker exclusion in Singapore'. *Identities*, 26(3): 356–73.

Humanitarian Organisation for Migrant Economics (HOME) and TWC2 (2010) *Justice Delayed, Justice Denied: The Experience of Migrant Workers in Singapore*. Singapore: HOME.

Kaur, S., Tan, N. and Dutta, M. (2016) 'Media, migration and politics: the coverage of the Little India riot in *The Straits Times*, Singapore'. *Journal of Creative Communications*, 11(1): 27–43.

Ministry of Manpower (2019) 'Foreign workforce numbers'. Retrieved from: www.mom.gov.sg/documents-and-publications/foreign-workforce-numbers

Opondo, S. and Shapino, M. (2020) 'Aesthetic separation/separation aesthetics: the pandemic and the event spaces of precarity'. *Geopolitica(s)*, 11: 223 8.

Transient Workers Count Too (TWC2) (2012) *NUS Students witness urban cleansing operation*. Retrieved from: https://twc2.org.sg/2012/11/06/nus-students-witness-cleansing-operation-against-foreign-workers/

Velayutham, R. (2009) 'Everyday racism in Singapore', in A. Wise and S. Velayutham (eds) *Everyday Multiculturalism*. London: Palgrave Macmillan, pp 255–73.

Ye, J. (2016) 'Spatializing the politics of urban co-existence: Gui Ju(规矩) in Singapore'. *Transactions of the Institute of British Geographers*, 41(1): 91–103.

Yea, S. (2017) 'The art of not being caught: temporal strategies for disciplining unfree labour in Singapore's contract migration'. *Geoforum*, 78: 179–88.

Yea, S. and Chok, S. (2018) 'Unfreedom unbound: developing a cumulative approach to understanding unfree labour in Singapore'. *Work, Employment and Society*, 32(5): 925–41.

PART IV

Age, Race, Gender, and Ability

Experiential Equity: An Environmental Neuroscientific Lens for Disparities in Urban Stress

Robin Mazumder

Urban stress

This pandemic has highlighted and demonstrated the bidirectional relationship between urban design and stress. At a very fundamental level, COVID-19, a communicable disease, has shifted how we engage with urban environments; places of connection that once brought joy may now be seen as places that expose us to threat of the disease. The term 'pandemic-related stress' refers to the stress and anxiety associated with contracting the illness, passing the illness onto others, as well as the financial stress associated with the pandemic's impact on the economy (Barzilay et al, 2020). As other chapters in this volume have emphasized, these impacts and their associated stresses vary considerably due to intersecting identities and geographies. There are many unknowns during the pandemic which have driven a sense of uncertainty and stress (Hirsch et al, 2012).

How, then, can we address this stress, which is a detrimental threat to central life goals? Considering that the threat of spreading, or contracting, the virus is primarily dependent on proximity to others within *indoor* spaces, the use of *outdoor* space, including both private and public spaces, could be seen as a way to mitigate pandemic-related stress. To help ensure the physical and mental well-being of residents, many cities have adapted their public spaces and built environments in order to increase the amount of open and public space available to use (see Volume 3). This has been done through the closing down of roadways to cars, implementing new bike lanes and, as more was learned about virus transmission, encouraging the use of park spaces. This outdoor-focused approach has been lauded as a necessary strategy to enhance and support physical and mental well-being (Mees, 2020; Mazumder, 2020). These open-air interventions, arguably, are also ways to help manage the perception and experience of the threat of contracting or spreading the virus. Furthermore, the exposure to greenspace has been found to be associated with a reduction in physiological measures of stress (Grahn and Stigsdotter, 2010). Access to, and experience of, public space, then, can be seen as a reliable and scalable solution to pandemic-related stress.

However, it is important to consider that not everyone experiences public space similarly, and that the pandemic is not the sole threat to safety (Beeckmans and Oosterlynck, Volume Three; Whitten and Massini, Volume Three; Rodriguez et al, Volume Three). In the midst of this pandemic, cities around the world have also erupted in protests highlighting the reality and pervasiveness of anti-Black racism. The pandemic and protests both involve a conversation about public space; while the pandemic has demonstrated the importance of how access to public space can support well-being, the protests demand we ask who that public space is open and accessible to. This chapter proposes a way of understanding how our intersectional identities play a major role in determining the different ways in which the same public spaces are accessed and experienced.

'Experiential equity' and differing experiences of the city

Planners, policy makers, city-builders, and advocates must therefore consider how equity applies to the experience of public space. This needs to be far more than box ticking or tokenism. Different experiences of the city need to be rooted in how urban spaces are planned, designed, and managed. In my own experience as a person of color, I can speak of the racist threats I've experienced in parks, and navigating streets and public spaces by foot and while on a bicycle. That said, I also recognize my privilege as a non–Black person of color, and that my experiences of public space differ based on my intersectional identity. The concept of intersectionality, first proposed by legal scholar Kimberlé Crenshaw (2018), is a helpful framework to examine the complexities and experiences of oppression in the urban context, because it acknowledges the multidimensionality of the human experience. Crenshaw highlights the ways in which discrimination associated with aspects of identity, including gender identity, gender, race, class, ability, and sexual orientation, intersect and amplify the experience of marginalization.

In the early 20th century, W.E.B. Du Bois, a Black sociologist, discussed twoness or double consciousness as a:

> sense of always looking at one's self through the eyes of others, of measuring one's soul by the tape of a world that looks on in amused contempt and pity. One ever feels his two-ness – an American, a Negro – two souls, two thoughts, two unreconciled strivings; two warring ideals in one dark body, whose dogged strength alone keeps it from being torn asunder. (Du Bois, 1903: 47)

This cognitive burden of racism, Double Consciousness, can be understood using Schmader et al's (2008) Integrated Model of Stereotype Threat, in which they propose that stereotype pressures have physiological stress consequences that affect working memory, which they define as 'a limited-capacity executive process that coordinates cognition and controls behavior to achieve performance goals in the presence of exogenous or endogenous information that competes for attention' (Schmader et al, 2008). Du Bois's Theory of Double Consciousness would suggest that racism, and the consequences it has on self-concept, constitutes the exogenous information (active experience of racism) and endogenous (anticipation of racism) information which is competing for cognitive resources. Furthermore, Clark et al (1999) proposed a biopsychosocial model of racism as a stressor to Black people, identifying the experience of racism as a cause of health disparities. This model builds on the stress-coping model originally proposed by Lazarus and Folkman (1984). They state that 'the perception of an environmental stimulus as racist results in exaggerated psychological and physiological stress responses that are influenced by constitutional factors, sociodemographic factors, psychological and behavioral factors, and coping responses' (Lazarus and Folkman, 1984: 806).

A consequence of this sustained and chronic racial stressor is the prolonged activation of the sympathetic nervous system (Clark et al, 1999). Hicken et al (2013) found that Black people reported higher levels of vigilance in daily activities compared to White and Hispanic people. Sewell et al (2016) further extend the impacts of racism on well-being, suggesting that police surveillance is a considerable contributor to racism-related vigilance. This is an incredibly important nuance that must be considered by environmental neuroscientists, particularly those who study urban environments, where racism is often perpetrated. Meyer (2003) proposes the concept of *minority stress*, which particularly acknowledges the stress of homophobia. However, within urban planning and urban studies, typical stressors rarely focus on race, racism, and discrimination, instead emphasizing factors such as noise, congestion, built environment variables, and crowding. As the pandemic places greater emphasis on public spaces, experiences such as racism, and other forms of systemic oppression, need to be considered a factor and a moderator of these pre-existing stressors.

Public space infrastructure that has been celebrated as a solution to well-being during this pandemic, such as cycling infrastructure and parks, is not, therefore, neutral space that is equally beneficial to everyone (see Scott, Volume Three; Mayers, Volume Four). As a result, the stress reduction benefits that have been attributed to parks and other public spaces may be negated by experiences of discrimination. To better understand the implications of this social climate on the physical parameters of urban environments, we can turn to the dominant environmental psychological theories of why greenspace is restorative. The dominant theories on the positive effects of greenspace requires that space to be unthreatening in order to be physiologically restorative (Ulrich et al, 1991; Kaplan, 1995). Therefore, it warrants questioning whether the threat of racism and other forms of oppression diminish the restorative benefits of nature? Furthermore, if being in public exposes one to racism or discrimination, or the fear of these experiences, can exposure to greenspace not only be non-beneficial, but actually detrimental to the emotional health of marginalized peoples?

This critical, intersectional lens is also relevant to cycling infrastructure's reported stress mitigating benefits. People who ride bicycles in cities prefer low traffic stress routes (Crist et al, 2019). Furth et al (2016) propose a model of levels of traffic stress, which positions vehicle traffic as the main form of stress. Separated cycling infrastructure, and its networked distribution, is suggested to reduce the level of stress a cyclist experiences, which can have effects on well-being. However, when we consider the implications of racism-related vigilance and minority stress, it would appear that cycling infrastructure alone will not ensure a stress-free ride for all cyclists. Again, we must acknowledge these disparities. Therefore, the popular and common planning and policy responses to the pandemic, such as the provision of new cycling infrastructure and greenspace will not be a solution to pandemic-related stress for everyone. The disparities of how these amenities are experienced must be considered. It is essential to recognize that we must simultaneously dismantle the systems which cause disparities in the experience of these amenities if we truly want everyone to benefit from them equally.

In their framework of urban green equity, Nesbitt et al (2019) propose distributional equity, which refers to spatial distribution of, and access to greenspace, and recognitional equity, which refers to the involvement of marginalized peoples in the park design decision process.

Building on these dimensions of urban equity, incorporating the Double Consciousness Theory (Du Bois, 1903), Intersectionality Theory (Crenshaw, 2018), Racism-Related Vigilance (Clark et al, 1999), and Minority Stress (Meyer, 2003), I propose the consideration of an *experiential equity*. Using my lens as an environmental neuroscientist, this term acknowledges the neurobiological, psychological, and behavioral disparities that exist in the human experience of public space, and the world at large, and the associated violence to the body and mind which are caused by these disparities. Experiential equity is a term that can help establish a measurable goal to achieve in public space that can be quantified using psychological and neuroscientific methods which can provide insight into the first-person experiences of inequitable spaces, and identify how these experiences influence the brain and the body. Considering the subjectivity of experiential equity, qualitative approaches will also be necessary in capturing the richness and diversity of experiences. To reiterate, the term *experiential equity* establishes that achieving equity is not solely about improving access to urban infrastructure, or its design or spatial distribution. Central to this concept is how one experiences that urban infrastructure. It applies a psychospatial lens to experiences of discrimination in public space.

Policy and practice implications

Using this approach to plan and evaluate urban spaces has taken on a greater sense of urgency because of the pandemic. Sanderson et al (2020) suggest that a main factor in pandemic-related stress is fear, which entails a perception of threat. This daily experience of threat is therefore amplified by the anticipation and experience of racism, and other forms of systemic oppression. This has implications for urban policy, planning, and practice. Using an experiential equity lens, it becomes clear that providing greenspace and infrastructure alone will not address the disparities that exist in our cities. To ensure a more equitable experience of these spaces, their planning, design, and governance must be centered in the *different* ways in which they are experienced. Intersectionality is essential. Jorgensen et al's (2013) focus on the fear women (can) experience in public space emphasized how increasing sightlines and visibility can help create a greater sense of safety in parks. This is an application of Jane Jacobs's (1961) assertion that 'eyes on the street' help make streets safer. However, given what is known about racism-related vigilance and its relationship to police surveillance, we must ask 'whose eyes and whose streets?' Again, an intersectional approach to these policies and design considerations is necessary to enhance our understanding of what safety means to different people, based on their unique identities, how they perceive their environments, and how they are perceived by others in these environments.

Urban design plays a role in eliminating disparities, and experiential equity is a lens that can be used to measure the improvement of outcomes. One spatial intervention using an intercultural lens to increase feelings of safety could involve incorporating public art that represents diverse communities in parks; Sharp et al (2005) suggest that public art can play a role in facilitating inclusion. A built environment that reflects the diversity of its users may appear to be more welcoming and intentionally inclusive. Further exploration into built environment interventions that can increase feelings of safety and a sense of welcoming is necessary; environmental neuroscience offers a methodology to objectively measure psychological and physiological effects of these interventions, and, consequently, the degree of experiential equity present in public space.

However, design alone will not address all of the barriers to experiential equity. We must also prioritize the dismantling of racist and oppressive systems that continue to perpetuate violence against marginalized communities. This entails a defunding of the police (see Dilworth and Weaver, Chapter Eighteen), an organization that creates feelings of fear for members of marginalized communities.

To ensure decision makers do not view equity as solely an issue of consultation, or spatial distribution of infrastructure, Experiential equity, and environmental neuroscience, must play a leading role in helping account for the diversity of experiences in our cities, using this knowledge to informing planning, policy, and design. Experiential equity centers gender identity, gender, race, class, ability, and sexual orientation in the different ways that we experience the same cities and urban spaces. As the pandemic has amplified the inequalities based around these identities, this approach is necessary to ensure everyone who lives in our cities benefits equally from urban infrastructure that supports well-being.

References

Barzilay, R., Moore, T.M., Greenberg, D.M., DiDomenico, G.E., Brown, L.A., White, L.K., Gur, R.C. and Gur, R.E. (2020) 'Resilience, COVID-19-related stress, anxiety and depression during the pandemic in a large population enriched for healthcare providers'. *Translational Psychiatry*, 10(1): 291.

Clark, R., Anderson, N.B., Clark, V.R. and Williams, D.R. (1999) 'Racism as a stressor for African Americans: a biopsychosocial model'. *The American Psychologist*, 54(10): 805–16.

Crenshaw, K. (2018) 'Demarginalizing the intersection of race and sex: a Black feminist critique of antidiscrimination doctrine, feminist theory, and antiracist politics' [1989], in *Feminist Legal Theory*, New York: Routledge, pp 57–80. https://doi.org/10.4324/9780429500480-5

Crist, K., Schipperijn, J., Ryan, S., Appleyard, B., Godbole, S. and Kerr, J. (2019) 'Fear factor: level of traffic stress and GPS assessed cycling routes'. *Journal of Transportation Technologies*, 9(1): 14–30. https://doi.org/10.4236/jtts.2019.91002

Du Bois, W.E.B. (1903) *The Souls of Black Folk*. New York: Penguin.

Furth, P.G., Mekuria, M.C. and Nixon, H. (2016) 'Network connectivity for low-stress bicycling'. *Transportation Research Record: Journal of the Transportation Research Board*, 2587(1): 41–9. https://doi.org/10.3141/2587-06

Grahn, P. and Stigsdotter, U.K. (2010) 'The relation between perceived sensory dimensions of urban green space and stress restoration'. *Landscape and Urban Planning*, 94(3–4): 264–75. https://doi.org/10.1016/j.landurbplan.2009.10.012

Hicken, M.T., Adar, S.D., Diez Roux, A.V., O'Neill, M.S., Magzamen, S., Auchincloss, A. H. and Kaufman, J.D. (2013) 'Do psychosocial stress and social disadvantage modify the association between air pollution and blood pressure? The multi-ethnic study of atherosclerosis'. *American Journal of Epidemiology*, 178(10): 1550–62.

Hirsh, J.B., Mar, R.A. and Peterson, J.B. (2012) 'Psychological entropy: a framework for understanding uncertainty-related anxiety'. *Psychological Review*, 119(2): 304–20.

Jacobs, J. (1961) *The Death and Life of Great American Cities*. New York: Random House.

Jorgensen, L.J., Ellis, G.D. and Ruddell, E. (2013) 'Fear perceptions in public parks: interactions of environmental concealment, the presence of people recreating, and gender'. *Environment and Behavior*, 45(7): 803–20.

Kaplan, S. (1995) 'The restorative benefits of nature: toward an integrative framework'. *Journal of Environmental Psychology*, 15(3): 169–82. https://doi.org/10.1016/0272-4944(95)90001-2

Lazarus, R.S. and Folkman, S. (1984) *Stress, Appraisal, and Coping.* New York: Springer Publishing Company.

Mazumder, R. (2020) 'Open parks and trust Canadians to social distance: we'll be healthier for it'. *Huffington Post*, April 16.

Mees, C. (2020) 'More shared urban open spaces: resiliency on demand'. *Agriculture and Human Values*, 37(3): 609–10.

Meyer, I.H. (2003) 'Prejudice, social stress, and mental health in lesbian, gay, and bisexual populations: conceptual issues and research evidence'. *Psychological Bulletin*, 129(5): 674.

Nesbitt, L., Meitner, M.J., Girling, C. and Sheppard, S.R.J. (2019) 'Urban green equity on the ground: practice-based models of urban green equity in three multicultural cities'. *Urban Forestry & Urban Greening*, 44: 126433. https://doi.org/10.1016/j.ufug.2019.126433

Sanderson, W.C., Arunagiri, V., Funk, A.P., Ginsburg, K.L., Krychiw, J.K., Limowski, A.R., Olesnycky, O.S. and Stout, Z. (2020) 'The nature and treatment of pandemic-related psychological distress'. *Journal of Contemporary Psychotherapy*, June 27: 1–13.

Schmader, T., Johns, M. and Forbes, C. (2008) 'An integrated process model of stereotype threat effects on performance'. *Psychological Review*, 115(2): 336–56.

Sewell, W., Horsford, C.E., Coleman, K. and Watkins, C.S. (2016) Vile vigilance: an integrated theoretical framework for understanding the state of Black surveillance'. *Journal of Human Behavior in the Social Environment*, 26(3–4): 287–302.

Sharp, J., Pollock, V. and Paddison, R. (2005) 'Just art for a just city: public art and social inclusion in urban regeneration'. *Urban Studies*, 42(5–6): 1001–23.

Ulrich, R.S., Simons, R.F., Losito, B.D., Fiorito, E., Miles, M.A. and Zelson, M. (1991) 'Stress recovery during exposure to natural and urban environments'. *Journal of Environmental Psychology*, 11(3): 201–30. https://doi.org/10.1016/s0272-4944(05)80184-7

What is the Relationship between COVID-19 and the Movement to 'Defund the Police'?

Richardson Dilworth and Timothy P.R. Weaver

COVID-19 triggered an extraordinary disruption to social, economic, and political life that is unprecedented in recent decades. As we have argued (in Dilworth and Weaver 2020), periods of major disruption give rise to unusually fluid circumstances in which settled political arrangements become vulnerable to assault by political entrepreneurs who promote radical ideas, hitherto marginal to the political debate. In such circumstances, those ideas can gain rapid traction and have the potential to drive political development. We suggest that the COVID-19 pandemic was one such disruption.

We argue in this chapter that pandemic-generated crises of political authority established the conditions for the 'defund the police' idea to shift from the fringes of political debate into the mainstream in the wake of George Floyd's murder at the hands of the police in May 2020. This is not to diminish the more fundamental causes for protest such as structural racism or police tyranny, but it seems possible that contingent factors, such as COVID-19, allowed Floyd's murder to become a unique catalyst that facilitated diffusion of the 'defund' idea across cities in the United States, and indeed across the world. Put simply, we suggest that amid the disarray into which the pandemic threw urban society, new social forces seized the opportunity to make demands that would have fallen on deaf ears in the absence of the disruptive effects of COVID-19. As such, it stands as a case study of the relationship between the pandemic and social movement politics.

Exploring the relationship between fundamental causes and contingent factors in the case of COVID-19 and the George Floyd killing allows us to better understand the dynamics of policy change. We start with a brief examination of the disruptions associated with COVID-19. We then explore the 'defund' idea and how it developed and diffused to specific cities. We finally consider how COVID-19 may have facilitated the diffusion of the idea, arguing that the relationship between the pandemic and the idea is more contingent and random than others have suggested, yet it also has the potential to significantly and permanently impact the trajectory of urban political development in the United States and beyond.

The great disruption

In February and March 2020 countries across the globe instituted a range of unprecedented limits on international travel, domestic movement of people, and mandated shutdowns of business and educational services to limit the spread of COVID-19. The social, political, and economic ramifications of these decisions were immediately felt and promise to last for years if not decades. We argue (building on a framework we developed in Dilworth and Weaver 2020) that the pandemic created profound instability and thus a context in which new ideas in general could have a greater reception. In certain contexts – namely liberal cities with large and more conservative but politically aggressive police departments – the idea that got the greatest reception was that to defund the police.

We started from the premise that new ideas have their greatest influence in times of crisis, instability, or disruption to the status quo, which overturn our settled assumptions and put us in search of new ideas, defined as explanations and propositions regarding how the world works. We further distinguished ideas from interests by arguing in part that, while interests are often defined on the basis of ideas, interests may then maintain their coherence in the absence of those ideas, either out of habit, some form of institutional path dependence, or some other reason. If older interests maintain their coherence in the presence of new ideas, those interests themselves will serve to maintain the strength of the older ideas, though those ideas may begin to look more like tribal beliefs, like clinging to symbols of a long-defeated nation such as the Confederate States of America, or to law enforcement needs defined during crime waves from the 1960s and 1970s.

Since major disruptions might differentially alter ideas and interests, we posited that new ideas would have the least influence in cases of low disruption to the status quo where existing interests maintained their coherence; indeterminate influence in cases of high disruption and high coherence, or low disruption but low coherence; and the greatest influence where disruptions were high and interests became incoherent. And COVID-19 clearly fits into the final category. By substantially altering the lives of practically every person on earth the pandemic has upended the daily rituals and routines through which our interests become internalized and thus institutionalized. By creating a zero-sum game between our financial and physical health the pandemic has also fundamentally disrupted our ability to cohesively define our interests – reflected, for instance, in public opinion polling indicating that the vast majority of Americans support social distancing and shelter-in-place policies (Kirzinger et al, 2020) even as they are more worried about the economy than about the health impacts of the virus (Butchireddygari, 2020) – aided and abetted by political leaders' contradictory and conflicted statements.

The pandemic might thus provide a context uniquely welcoming of new ideas, but what ideas? Where will these ideas come from? Where are they most likely to be adopted? To answer these questions we started with two basic assumptions – that big cities are distinct from the larger society, and also disruptive places uniquely capable of generating and adopting new ideas – from which we derived three potential paths of diffusion, all of which start with new ideas generated in one or a few big cities, which then (1) diffuse across the larger society but not to other big cities; (2) diffuse across the larger society, including to big cities; and (3) diffuse to other big cities but not the larger society.

The history and geography of an idea

The idea to defund police departments was developed and sustained by left activist and academic networks from the 1960s that became more focused in the 1990s around the increasing incarceration rate, the growth of private prisons, and increasing police budgets, now known collectively as the 'carceral state'. The movement to dismantle the carceral state has been termed one of 'abolition', implying a trajectory that connects slavery to the contemporary disproportionate policing and imprisonment of Black Americans.

The most prominent abolitionist organizations are typically located in larger cities and college towns. Thus, for instance, the abolitionist and Ohio State University law professor Amna Akbar (2020), in a recent and brief historical survey of the abolitionist movement, mentions groups in Minneapolis, Berkeley, Oakland, New York, Los Angeles, Portland (Oregon), Detroit, Atlanta, St. Louis, Chicago, Seattle, and Durham (North Carolina). A highly influential publication from abolitionist activist groups that documented increasing police department expenditures – *Freedom to Thrive* (2017) – was written 'in collaboration with 27 local organizations around the country' (2017: i), all of which are headquartered in either New York City, Los Angeles, Chicago, St. Louis, Detroit, the Minneapolis-St Paul twin cities, Atlanta (or an Atlanta suburb), San Francisco, Oakland, Baltimore, Phoenix, Miami, or Orlando.

The available evidence suggests a substantial overlap between cities with strong activist networks and those where officials are seriously considering or have already adopted new policies related to the defund idea, including actually disbanding a police force, decreasing police department budgets, redirecting 911 calls to social service agencies, or setting up a task force to study the issue. For instance, of the 17 cities mentioned by Akbar (2020) or who contributed to *Freedom to Thrive*, nine were also identified in early journalistic efforts to catalog cities in which officials had acted on or were seriously considering 'defund'-related ideas (Holder, 2020; McEvoy, 2020).

Including the cities identified by journalists but not by Akbar or included in *Freedom to Thrive* (San Diego; Dallas; Austin; Philadelphia; Salt Lake City; Washington, D.C.; Hartford, Connecticut; and Norman, Oklahoma) provides for a total list of 25 cities. Among the features that unite most of these cities is that they are typically racially and ethnically diverse; 11 are less than half White, and all but Portland and Norman have a lower percentage of White people than the US overall, which is 76.3 percent White (though Miami, Phoenix, Austin, and Salt Lake City come very close, at 75 percent, 72 percent, 74 percent, and 73 percent, respectively). Similarly, 14 of these cities have a higher percent Black population than the US overall (13.4 percent), and every city has a higher percentage of people in poverty, with the exceptions of Seattle (which falls right at the overall US rate of 11.8 percent) and San Francisco (10.9 percent).

Yet possibly the most significant element that unites each of these cities is that they are all majority Democratic, as indicated by the fact that all but two have (as of September 2020) Democratic mayors, and even in the cases of Miami and San Diego where there are Republican mayors, there are more registered Democrats than Republicans. The overwhelming Democratic identity of big-city dwellers is of course old news, as numerous polls have shown that the yawning partisan divide in the US is also a geographic divide between urban and ex- or nonurban areas.

Notably, one group of big-city employees who are least likely to be Democrats are the police. Their national union, the Fraternal Order of Police (FOP), endorsed Donald Trump for president in 2016, and a 2016 email poll in *Police* magazine found that 84 percent of the 3,652 respondents said that they planned to vote for Trump (Griffith, 2016). Moreover, most big-city police, especially if they are White, do not actually live in the cities where they work – of the 25 cities examined here, only Chicago, St Louis, and Hartford require that police live in the city, and even in those cities residency requirements are often ignored – only slightly more than half of St Louis police officers actually live in St Louis, for instance (Ungar-Sargon and Flowers, 2014; Silver, 2014).

In short, the likelihood that the 'defund' idea will diffuse across cities is conditioned by the unique circumstances of activist networks and Democratic city officials who oversee large police budgets, combined with police who typically do not live in the city, are more conservative, and more White than city residents, but who are politically active in the city through FOP lobbying and fundraising (Perkins, 2020). Moreover, the 'defund' idea is itself vague and thus flexible, which makes it amenable to less radical interpretations that can be embraced by local politicians – as we have noted elsewhere, the flexibility of most ideas allows them to operate as 'emulsifiers that allow actors to blend otherwise disparate and potentially incompatible elements into a definition of a new world order defined by new institutional arrangements' (Dilworth and Weaver, 2020: 12).

For instance, Minneapolis, where Floyd was murdered, has a vibrant abolitionist activist network, and it was the Minneapolis city council that took the most dramatic step of voting by a veto-proof majority to disband the city's police department and replace it with a 'Department of Community Safety and Violence Prevention', which would ostensibly still include law enforcement but focus more on alternate means of maintaining public order and safety. (The measure requires a charter change and thus approval by referendum, which has been blocked until at least 2021.) Mayor Jacob Frey opposed disbanding the police but has also used the controversy to revisit contract negotiations with the FOP. As one former Minneapolis council member put it, 'The more public the city's desires are, the more pressure there will be on the Police Department that has become out of step' (quoted in Forliti, 2020). In short, Minneapolis's mayor and council may disagree on the shape of police reform, but the council has effectively played 'bad cop' for the mayor, allowing him greater leverage in union negotiations.

How are the 'defund' idea and COVID-19 related?

Abolitionist activist networks and Democratic city officials have lived with conservative and politically aggressive police departments for many years; yet only during the COVID-19 pandemic did the 'defund' idea gain traction. What is the specific connection between COVID-19 and the diffusion of the 'defund' idea? One explanation is simply that the pandemic-induced economic depression has reduced city and state government budgets, with the result that police budgets would have to be cut. As one New York state senator noted in response to New York City mayor Bill DeBlasio's attempts to maintain a $6 billion budget for the New York Police Department, 'Having come out of a bleak state budget process, it's very frustrating to hear that $6bn figure for the NYPD' (quoted in Levin, 2020).

Budget shortfalls may explain incremental budget cuts but not the rapid diffusion of the idea to defund the police – even as that idea has provided leverage for instituting incremental budget cuts. An alternate explanation is that COVID-19 has exacerbated the effects of racism and thus made racist and deadly police actions more consequential. As Levin (2020) put it, 'The unconscionable examples of racism over the last weeks and months come as America's communities of color have been hit hardest by the coronavirus and catastrophic job losses.' Yet this also does not explain the impact of the 'defund' idea in cities with small Black populations, such as Portland, Seattle, Salt Lake City, Norman, and Phoenix. Moreover, it seems unlikely that most Americans, who are White, would be fully aware of the racially disproportionate impact of COVID-19 – yet a majority of Americans in July reported in polls that they thought 'major changes' in policing were needed, even if most did not support police abolition itself (Crabtree, 2020).

Finally, political scientist LaGina Gause (2020) has argued that policy makers are more responsive when protestors risk more for their cause. The possibility of infection made protesting riskier, thereby ostensibly making policy makers more amenable to protestor demands such as defunding the police. Yet the economic shutdown also means that many protestors are not sacrificing or risking their wages or jobs by spending time on the frontlines, which made protesting arguably easier and, at least in an economic sense, less risky.

What these explanations all have in common is that they suggest the pandemic itself created greater support for defunding the police, or at least for police reform. By contrast, we maintain here that the pandemic's general effect was to create deep instability, especially in places where the radical ideas such as defunding the police were likely to gain the most traction. The 'defund' idea originated primarily among activist networks in larger American cities and diffused to other larger cities, but hardly anywhere else. A case in point is Texas, where the state's four largest cities (Houston, Dallas, San Antonio, and

Austin) have all faced pressure to defund the police, and have all seriously considered the proposal. The Austin City Council went the furthest in voting to cut its police department budget by $150 million. Yet in a reflection of quite different sentiment outside the big cities, GOP state legislators have proposed to freeze the property tax rates of any city that cut police budgets, and in early 2021, the governor is currently and very publicly investigating a potential state takeover of the Austin police.

Texas, though possibly a somewhat extreme case, exemplifies a broader pattern of increasing partisan polarization between urban and nonurban areas, reflected as well *within* cities between police and more liberal residents and elected officials. That partisan context is one in which COVID-19 served as a catalyst for policy change unique to big cities that has further exacerbated the partisan divide between big cities and the rest of American society, possibly to enough of an extent that this urban-nonurban partisan and ideological divide has become qualitatively broader and more permanent.

References

Akbar, A.A. (2020) 'How defund and disband became the demands'. *The New York Review*, June 16. www.nybooks.com/daily/2020/06/15/how-defund-and-disband-became-the-demands/

Butchireddygari, L. (2020) 'Americans are worried about the coronavirus. They're even more worried about the economy'. *Five Thirty Eight*, March 27. https://fivethirtyeight.com/features/americans-are-worried-about-the-coronavirus-theyre-even-more-worried-about-the-economy/

Crabtree, S. (2020) 'Most Americans say policing needs "major changes"'. *Gallup*, July 22. https://news.gallup.com/poll/315962/americans-say-policing-needs-major-changes.aspx

Dilworth, R. and Weaver, T.P.R. (2020) 'Ideas, interests, institutions, and urban political development', in R. Dilworth and T.P.R. Weaver (eds) *How Ideas Shape Urban Political Development*. Philadelphia: University of Pennsylvania Press, pp 1–18.

Forliti, A. (2020) 'Minneapolis leaders push ahead with efforts to change police'. *The Washington Post*, August 6. www.washingtonpost.com/health/minneapolis-leaders-push-ahead-with-efforts-to-change-police/2020/08/06/0b277822-d84b-11ea-a788-2ce86ce81129_story.html

Freedom to Thrive: Reimagining Safety and Security in Our Communities (2017) New York: Center for Popular Democracy.

Gause, L. (2020) 'Black people have protested police killings for years. Here's why officials are finally responding'. *The Washington Post*, June 12. www.washingtonpost.com/politics/2020/06/12/black-people-have-protested-police-killings-years-heres-why-officials-are-finally-responding/

Griffith, D. (2016) 'The 2016 POLICE presidential poll'. *Police*, September 2. www.policemag.com/342098/the-2016-police-presidential-poll

Holder, S. (2020) 'The cities taking up calls to defund the police'. Bloomberg City Lab, June 9. www.bloomberg.com/news/articles/2020-06-09/the-cities-taking-up-calls-to-defund-the-police

Kirzinger, A., Hamel, L., Muñana, C., Kearney, A. and Brodie, M. (2020). 'Coronavirus, social distancing, and contact tracing'. *Kaiser Family Foundation*, April 24. www.kff.org/global-health-policy/issue-brief/kff-health-tracking-poll-late-april-2020/

Levin, S. (2020) 'Movement to defund police gains "unprecedented" support across US'. *The Guardian*, June 4. www.theguardian.com/us-news/2020/jun/04/defund-the-police-us-george-floyd-budgets

McEvoy, J. (2020) 'At least 13 cities are defunding their police departments'. *Forbes*, August 13. www.forbes.com/sites/jemimamcevoy/2020/08/13/at-least-13-cities-are-defunding-their-police-departments/#2c32562429e3

Perkins, T. (2020) 'Revealed: police unions spend millions to influence policy in biggest US cities'. *The Guardian*, June 23. www.theguardian.com/us-news/2020/jun/23/police-unions-spending-policy-reform-chicago-new-york-la

Silver, N. (2014) 'Most police don't live in the cities they serve'. *Five Thirty Eight*, August 20. https://fivethirtyeight.com/features/most-police-dont-live-in-the-cities-they-serve/

Ungar-Sargon. B. and Flowers, A. (2014) 'Reexamining residency requirements for police officers'. *Five Thirty Eight*, October 1. https://fivethirtyeight.com/features/reexamining-residency-requirements-for-police-officers/

Following the Voices of Older Adults During the COVID-19 Crisis: Perspectives from the Netherlands

Jolanda Lindenberg, Paul van de Vijver, Lieke de Kock,

David van Bodegom, and Niels Bartels

Introduction

COVID-19 has impacted our lives suddenly and drastically. From the first cases in China to the millions infected worldwide, attention has focused on those at highest risk of adverse health outcomes: older adults. Yet similarly striking was the lack of attention given to the actual voices of older adults (see Hartt et al, Volume Four; Osborne et al, Volume Three; Low and Loukaitou-Sideris, Volume Three). This is despite previous research having shown that disregarding the voices of older adults in disaster situations may lead to increased anxiety, decreased self-efficacy, and post-crisis stress (Campbell, 2019). Recent COVID-19 studies that pay attention to older people are overwhelmingly based on quantitative, survey-based research. Although very valuable, limited attention is paid to the heterogeneity among older adults. To uncover the diverse voices about experiences during the COVID-19 pandemic among older individuals, their close relatives, and people involved in their care, we developed the website www. wijencorona.nl, which translates as 'Corona and us.' On this platform, experiences are shared, primarily by older Dutch individuals, but also by people from other countries and younger individuals.

The Dutch government implemented an 'intelligent' lockdown, starting in March, 2020 (Antonides and van Leeuwen, 2020). This approach to managing the pandemic appealed to solidarity and self-discipline in order to comply with social distancing, and staying at home as much as possible. Essential shops and services remained open, and people were allowed to go out when deemed necessary, unlike in other countries, such as France. During this 'intelligent' lockdown and the pandemic's first wave (March–May 2020), almost 250 people from four different continents shared their stories on our website. Each contribution averaged around 700 words, providing rich detail and examples of life during the pandemic. In this chapter, we focus only on the stories shared by individuals aged 50 years and older, which by June 2020, comprised a total of 191 individuals. We present four examples – Mbarek, Joke, Wim, and Maria – that represent the broader discourses and experiences found throughout this project as we explored and analyzed the voices of older adults during the first wave of COVID-19 in the Netherlands (for a similar approach, see Rocco et al, Chapter Twelve). More specifically, we delve into their views of experiencing COVID-19 in an urban or rural context. We draw upon these stories to discover opportunities for rural and urban futures.

'It's a strange sensation'

In the Netherlands, mitigation measures focused on hygiene, avoiding social contact, and staying at home as much as possible.

Lockdown measures were implemented swiftly in March 2020. Illustratively, on March 9, 2020 the Prime Minister advised against shaking hands and emphasized that more stringent measures were not necessary. To great amusement, he then shook hands on camera with the medical expert standing next to him! Just three days later, on March 12, 2020, he had to announce more stringent measures. On that day, the whole country was advised to stay at home and avoid social contact. These first measures were quickly expanded towards the 'intelligent' lockdown (see Kuiper et al, 2020) that lasted until May 6, 2020. It is therefore no surprise that older adults on the Wijencorona website focused on the rapid and unexpected changes in their lives. They felt taken off guard with how suddenly their lives were disrupted. The way they situated and interpreted this was diverse. In Table 19.1, we highlight four stories from rural and urban contexts. For some, this change was something they had to live through, and for others it generated fear and uncertainty, especially in assessing their individual risk. This is particularly the case for Joke. As a consequence of her low literacy, her anxiety was fueled by her inability to fully understand what was going on and what would keep her safe. She stated: 'By now, my hands are totally rough and ripped because of all the handwashing. I wash them continuously throughout the day. On television, they've said to wash your hands more. I do that.'

'From approaching to avoiding'

In Table 19.2, the four individuals described how they experienced the effects of the lockdown. Irrespective of whether they lived in a rural or urban setting, social distancing greatly affected their daily lives. Social contacts, daily activities, and grocery shopping were now about how to avoid people. As Wim described, interactions shifted 'from approaching to avoiding'. Maria, Wim, and others spent their time differently, such as by doing puzzles, reading, or other

Table 19.1: Situating COVID-19

Name (pseudonym)	Age, marital status, urban or rural	Quotations
Mbarek	70, married, city	'The first seven weeks were very quiet.'
Joke	68, widow, city	'It's so boring. I don't see anyone. In the beginning, I totally didn't understand. I heard things on television and I thought: "What do they mean?" I got nervous, got pain in my stomach, and had to throw up. I didn't feel like living and stopped eating and cooking.'
Wim	73, LAT relation, (temporary) rural	'It is intense what is happening, but I don't feel it that way [worrying] yet.'
Maria	70, married, rural	'It is a strange sensation that I turned 70 and belong to the high-risk group, while I am in good health and feel safe in that sense.'

Source: authors

leisure activities. Joke and Mbarek described how their lives were boring or less meaningful. The way they organized their social distancing did not differ much between urban and rural contexts, but Wim, Maria, and others on the platform felt that in rural settings it was easier to keep one's distance and it was therefore safer than in big cities. Wim, for example, chose to move in with his girlfriend, who lived in a small village, in order to be together and avoid the busy city. Maria, who also resided in a rural setting, also felt she was on a 'safe island'. The reasoning she gave for this was that being close to nature would reduce her risk because it felt easier to avoid people. However, in the Netherlands,

Table 19.2: Dealing with the COVID-19 crisis

Name	Age and status	Living	Groceries	Daily life	Social contacts	(In)formal care/ caregiving
Mbarek	70, married, city	'Now we have been home for months. We didn't go anywhere.'	'Groceries were brought to us, or, very seldomly, my wife went to the supermarket.'	'The thing that I miss the most about my daily routine: going to the gym, the library and, with a group older migrants, I teach via the foundation the Emigration generation at primary schools in Utrecht. That is a lot of fun.'	'The kids and grandchildren regularly visit. They stand in front of the window and that's how we talk. [...] I don't participate in Ramadan because I am diabetic. We celebrated Eid al Fitr. Very small, without children and grandchildren, but we did have lots of tasty food.'	'Once, I joined my wife in the car and went to see the kids. The grandchildren didn't understand this at all: "Why do grandpa and grandma stay in the car and why don't they come in?" We will not be doing that again.'

(continued)

Table 19.2: Dealing with the COVID-19 crisis (continued)

Name	Age and status	Living	Groceries	Daily life	Social contacts	(In)formal care/ caregiving
Joke	68, widow, city	'I don't see anyone. Both my daughters work. One in an office supplies store and the other is a train conductor. They are in contact with so many people, I don't dare to get close to them. [...] Now I am at home or on the balcony. I don't go out of my apartment, because it would be impossible to sit in the park where I might contract who knows what, while not seeing my girls at the same time.'	'Now, my daughter does it and I have to write it down and read it to my daughter. I write it down in my own way and if my daughter calls I try to read it aloud. Last week, we were on the phone for an hour, because I can't read what I wrote myself. Luckily she says: "Mom, take it slow, I have time."'	'It is so boring. [...] Before COVID-19, Conny and Joyce from "Stembevrijders" [liberators of voice] dropped by every month with singing bowls. That is so lovely, it completely relaxes me. Hopefully I will see them again this year, because I miss them tremendously.'	'I have told my girls that we may be able to only see each other at the end of November and that it might not ever be like before. What is life then? How should it continue?'	'My home help still visits every week. The way it goes is very strange. She is in the living room, then I go to the bedroom, and when she does the bedroom then I have to go to the living room. That is how she prefers to do it. She visits so many people at home and doesn't want to infect me. She doesn't wear gloves or

(continued)

Table 19.2: Dealing with the COVID-19 crisis (continued)

Name	Age and status	Living	Groceries	Daily life	Social contacts	(In)formal care/ caregiving
						a face mask, and that scares me. But also what should I do?' her stories, when she tells me what she has done in the past week I think to myself: where did you go? What if you are infected? At night I wake up and I think to myself: what if she wouldn't visit any more? I won't manage alone, what should I do?'

(continued)

Table 19.2: Dealing with the COVID-19 crisis (continued)

Name	Age and status	Living	Groceries	Daily life	Social contacts	(In)formal care/ caregiving
Wim	73, LAT relation, (temporary) rural	'My girlfriend Christine and I have a long-distance relation[ship]. Normally, we alternate between a long weekend at my place in the city and her[s] in a village. Now, I am at her place a lot, because she has several chronic diseases and is extra vulnerable. You better avoid the city then. Now and then we go to the city so I can check everything at home.	'We order our groceries from the supermarket in the village, [and] we can pick them up in crates at a delivery point. So we don't have to go into the store.'	'We are very rural here, at the edge of the village. Five minutes from the countryside. Every afternoon, we walk about two to three hours through nature. [...] At home, we make sure to maintain a good rhythm and structure in the day, so we remain in cadence. We play board games. We do puzzles and watch televisions. In the garden we watch the birds.'	'Everything I did has ceased. [...] We kind of live a hermit's life, we avoid contact with other people. From approaching to avoiding behavior, that is kind of alienating.'	

(continued)

Table 19.2: Dealing with the COVID-19 crisis (continued)

Name	Age and status	Living	Groceries	Daily life	Social contacts	(In)formal care/ caregiving
Maria	70, married, rural	'The past week I stayed home. [...] In our own home, I feel pretty safe. That's also because we have a large house, with a large garden around it and with few people in the direct neighborhood. It kind of feels like you're on a safe island. On top of that, we live in a small village in the south of Limburg where it's always quiet.'	'My husband does the groceries, but now at a moment when the shop is quiet.'	'But on the other hand, I can keep myself busy with reading, crochet, and the iPad. I don't manage to do the things I would normally not get to. I have not started cleaning the house. But who knows, that might still happen.'	'Sadly, I cannot participate in my normal social activities such as line dancing, painting classes, and two choirs; I find that unfortunate[.] I don't find it too bad to stay at home. What I do find a pity is that I cannot visit our grandson in Amsterdam. Luckily, we have FaceTime.'	

Source: authors

rates of infection were highest in rural areas during the first weeks of the pandemic, in contrast to some other countries (see Boterman, 2020). The first outbreaks and hotspots were centered in Noord-Brabant, a province with a population density of 522/km^2 (in contrast, Noord-Holland, the province where Amsterdam is situated, is the most densely populated province, at 1081/km^2 (CBS, 2020)). The first case in Noord-Brabant appeared during Carnaval, a major regional festival. In March 2020, three villages and small communities in Noord-Brabant had the highest infection rates of any Dutch municipality: Boekel: 10,588 inhabitants, Uden: 41,782 inhabitants, and Bernheze: 30,432 inhabitants. Analyses of the spread of COVID-19 in the Netherlands actually showed that the risk of infection was related to the density of bonds within a certain locale, irrespective of it being an urban or rural setting, rather than the number of people per square kilometer.

Besides perceived levels of safety, this rural 'imaginary' signified relaxation and freedom. Especially prominent were stories about walking in nature (or in parks) during which one was free to roam around. The allure of nature is also evidenced by soaring rates of visitors to natural areas (Nu.nl, 2020). Thus, nature played an additional role in providing a sense of freedom, particularly when other freedoms were taken away.

As is clear from the descriptions, not everyone started this crisis with the same resources and opportunities. Joke's story in particular demonstrates a magnification of her vulnerability through intersecting disadvantages. These included being on a low income, residing in a small home with little outdoor space and few opportunities to find alternatives. Yet Joke still managed; she asked for help within her social network, and later she found help with a support hotline. She also shared her voice and her story on the website. And people responded; she received gifts, cards, flowers, and balloons which decreased her feelings of isolation. She was seen and acknowledged. Even though she managed, importantly this was not because of the resources her environment provided, but despite the resources.

More considerate

The COVID-19 crisis is specific, as in this disaster is not so much about the dangerous aspects of certain spaces (such as safety, or living in an earthquake prone area), but about the risk of meeting someone and contracting the virus from that exchange. In the voices of older adults, urban or rural characteristics were of less importance than the social distancing that they can, and are, willing to uphold. This seems easier in less densely populated rural areas that geographically have more space. But as is also known, nodes in urban networks are usually more fragmented and less dense, and perhaps in this crisis less risky. However, for the feeling of self-determination and individual freedom actual space is highlighted in the stories of older adults. It is the voices of these older individuals that we followed in what, according to them, has priority, namely that, as Wim describes, in the future: 'I expect us to become more considerate, more focused on others. A larger societal engagement.' Or as Maria says, 'Might COVID-19 change that and lead to different behavior? Less materialistic and more social?' Their priorities overwhelmingly lie with social engagement and connections in their lives. Spaces, whether urban or rural, should be taken as their priority. If we consider potential urban futures, as futures in which older adults live well, we need to focus on how these urban settings allow for connections with relatives, with neighbors, with others, because it is the lack thereof that is missed the most during COVID-19.

Conclusion

It is often assumed that social avoidance is difficult in urban settings. This may be the case, but given the way COVID-19 spread in the Netherlands initially, it was not so much the density of people but rather sheer coincidence (a large regional festival) and the density of networks of people that mattered (see also Hoekman et al, 2020). As such, urban settings were perhaps less risky than rural settings. However, perhaps equally important, the way rural spaces allowed for social distancing made older adults feel less at risk in more rural areas. Nature gave them a sense of freedom and self-determination. Irrespective of urban or rural setting, opportunities for societal engagement were missed the most. For a crisis that can only be solved through social distancing, this is an inherent dilemma. Listening to the voices of older adults, we have to find ways to make sure that the (built) environment enables social engagement and interaction as we move into new phases of the pandemic. Besides this rather unequivocal theme, stories of older adults indicate that we should take into account the heterogeneity among older individuals and the diverse ways they situate, cope with, and interpret the crisis. It draws our attention, yet again, to how crises magnify vulnerabilities and lead some to experience intersecting difficulties. Acknowledging this heterogeneity is something that is necessary not just in times of crisis.

The voices in this chapter also highlight how we mainly talk *about* and decide *for* older adults, *instead* of with them. Additionally, we often approach this segment of the population as one homogeneous group through (unconscious) ageist attitudes (Staudinger, 2015). Combating this ageist inclination should be one of the highest priorities in the next decade as these can be detrimental for the experience of aging, health, and social participation (Officer and de la Fuente-Núñez, 2018). As such, changing the built and social environment according to the priorities of older adults – focusing on enabling social engagement – is not just a choice in urban planning and design, but can contribute to the position of older adults and the way we perceive aging.

References

Antonides, G. and van Leeuwen, E. (2020) 'Covid-19 crisis in the Netherlands: "Only together we can control Corona"'. *Mind & Society*, 1–7. https://doi.org/10.1007/s11299-020-00257-x

Boterman, W. (2020) 'Urban-rural polarisation in times of the Corona outbreak? The early demographic and geographic patterns of the SARS-CoV-2 epidemic in the Netherlands'. *Tijdschrift voor economische en sociale geografie*, 111(3) (July): 513–29. https://doi.org/10.1111/tesg.12437

Campbell, N. (2019) 'Disaster recovery among older adults: exploring the intersection of vulnerability and resilience', in F.I. Rivera (ed) *Emerging Voices in Natural Hazards Research*. Oxford: Butterworth-Heinemann, pp 83–119. https://doi.org/10.1016/B978-0-12-815821-0.00011-4

CBS (2020) 'Composition of the population on January 1, 2020'. https://opendata.cbs.nl/#/CBS/nl/dataset/70072ned/table?ts=1619643112941

Hoekman, L.M., Smits, M.M.V. and Koolman, X. (2020) 'The Dutch COVID-19 approach: regional differences in a small country'. *Health Policy and Technology*, 9(4): 613–22. DOI: 10.1016/j.hlpt.2020.08.008

Kuiper, M.E., de Bruijn, A.L., Reinders Folmer, C., Olthuis, E., Brownlee, M., Kooistra, E.B., Fine, A. and van Rooij, B. (2020) 'The intelligent lockdown: compliance with COVID-19 mitigation measures in the Netherlands'. *SSRN Electronic Journal*. https://doi.org/10.2139/ssrn.3598215

Nu.nl (2020) *Nederlanders gaan massaal de natuur in vanwege coronavirus [Dutch massively visit nature because of Covid-19]*. March 17. www.nu.nl/coronavirus/6038153/nederlanders-gaan-massaal-de-natuur-in-vanwege-coronavirus.html

Officer, A. and de la Fuente-Núñez, V. (2018) 'A global campaign to combat ageism'. *Bulletin World Health Organization*, 96(4): 295–6. DOI: 10.2471/BLT.17.202424

Staudinger, U.M. (2015) 'Images of aging: outside and inside perspectives'. *Annual Review of Gerontology and Geriatrics*, 35(1): 187–209. DOI: 10.1891/0198-8794.35.187

The Role of Social Infrastructures for Trans* People During the COVID-19 Pandemic

Magdalena Rodekirchen and Sawyer Phinney

The relationship of lesbian, gay, bisexual, transgender, and queer (LGBTQ) people and cities, and the urban geography of queerness, has been well documented in scholarly literature (Doderer, 2011; Gieseking, 2015). Cities are vital to the LGBTQ movement, and most key activism has taken place in urban centers over the last several decades. In comparison to rural areas, cities serve as spaces of difference. Moreover, the suburbs and suburbanization brought a 're-norming' of the heterosexual family which often made it essential for LGBTQ people to concentrate in cities (Gieseking, 2015: 15). Queering urban spaces has been carried out, resisted, and performed through social infrastructures that have contributed to the establishment of LGBTQ communities by 'defining themselves via voluntary kinship, social and cultural life (and indeed political demands)' (Doderer, 2011: 434). Drawing on the concept of social infrastructure (see also Auerbach et al, Chapter Eleven), we outline the ways in which the urban inequities of transgender and gender non-conforming people (trans* people) have changed because of the COVID-19 pandemic. We situate trans* people's urban inequities against the backdrop of UK austerity cuts which have undermined social infrastructures vital to LGBTQ communities. We argue that due to these pre-existing conditions, trans* people are disproportionately affected by the pandemic in terms of social infrastructures of health, community, and housing.

Social infrastructures

A recent 'infrastructural turn' (Amin, 2014) has seen increased attention being paid to infrastructures as a relational concept, as the sociotechnical systems that co-constitute the possibilities of social life in urban spaces. Infrastructures both inscribe and order difference, marginalizing and excluding gendered bodies and ways of being that differ from hegemonic norms of masculinity scripted into infrastructural workings (Siemiatycki et al, 2020: 1). Social infrastructures include places, such as community buildings, in which people can interact, form relationships, and create a sense of community. People play a vital role in social infrastructures, as articulated in Simone's concept of 'people as infrastructure', which draws attention to people's activities of community organizing in a city (Simone, 2004: 407). Community spaces and the people's activities that maintain them are particularly important for sustaining social life in the UK, where austerity following 2008 has resulted in severe cuts to public services, undermining social infrastructures. As a consequence of these cuts, the burden has been increasingly placed on non-state actors and organizations to fill in the gap.

Building on personal and intimate geographies of austerity, that is, the ways in which austerity seeps into personal, family lives, and networks (Hall, 2015), a recent intervention by Sarah Hall (2020) extends debates on social infrastructures beyond their understanding as 'community-building in community buildings' to social reproduction as infrastructural. As Wilson (2016) and later Datta and Ahmed (2020) argue, infrastructures are intimate and deeply gendered, both with regard to their impacts and the possibilities of navigating within them. However, Hall (2020: 91) reminds us that even beyond these gendered dynamics 'at the heart of the concept of social infrastructure (even if it is taken, as a minimum, to entail community venues and social spaces) is gendered, reproductive labour'. A strong emphasis on the role of physical infrastructures risks making invisible the 'processes, practices and people that maintain and sustain its existence' (Hall, 2020: 91). Drawing on feminist framings of social reproduction as the labor that allows societies to function, Hall (2020) conceptualizes social reproduction as a form of infrastructure that, through gendered labor at multiple scales, enables societies to function. In this way, social infrastructure is social reproduction where social relations are inextricably embedded into the workings of material infrastructures. The important role of community ties to the social reproduction of transgender and gender non-conforming people, that we understand as a form of social infrastructure, has become particularly visible during the COVID-19 pandemic.

Building on these debates, we posit that even before COVID-19, the gendered inequities of austerity cuts to public services have had a particularly harmful impact on trans* people in the UK, heightening the vital importance of social infrastructures for their day-to-day survival. With the onset of the pandemic, many of the social relations and invisible labor that underlie social infrastructures broke down, placing trans* people in a particularly precarious position. For the remainder of the chapter, we aim to tease out the specific inequities experienced by trans* people in the UK during the first wave of the COVID-19 pandemic, drawing on social infrastructures as a conceptual lens.

Urban inequities of transgender people and social infrastructures

Even though rural spaces are not sexually monolithic, a higher prevalence of hate crimes against LGBTQ people in general and trans* people in particular in Britain's rural towns and villages (Hardy and Chakraborti, 2015) can be linked to a queer migration pattern, particularly among youth, towards established urban LGBTQ communities and spaces, such as Brighton, Manchester, and London. Such urban communities provide access to LGBTQ organizations and support networks, including for mental and physical health, housing, and community spaces.

To better understand how the pandemic has accelerated inequities in social infrastructures for trans* people residing in urban locations, we systematically reviewed existing research on the impact of COVID-19 on LGBTQ communities, as well as newspaper articles and reports, including the LGBT Foundation's COVID-19 report of LGBT people living in the UK, which is based on a community online survey and service user data (LGBT Foundation, 2020). Based on our data collected between April and September 2020 and our preliminary findings of COVID-19 impacts on LGBTQ people, we identified three main social infrastructures that are fundamental to the social reproduction of trans* individuals but have been made vulnerable during the pandemic. These include health care, community belonging, and housing.

Social infrastructures of health

Prior to the onset of COVID-19, trans* people already faced significant barriers to access gender affirming care due to government funding cuts, gatekeeping, and discrimination. For example, trans* people, in particular Black and trans* People of Color, are more likely to experience discrimination by medical staff or not receive appropriate treatment (Kattari et al,

2016). With COVID-19, most health care providers canceled, or indefinitely postponed surgeries classified as non-necessary, including gender-affirming surgeries (such as mastectomies or genital reassignment surgeries). Even though a range of surgeries classified as non-essential were postponed indefinitely to increase capacity of health services for COVID-19 in-patient care, the very classification of gender-affirming surgeries as non-essential in primo loco warrants particular attention. Such a re-classification of trans*-surgeries can be traced back to the idea that these procedures are based on a desire for *aesthetical* change (as opposed to *life-saving*) and therefore non-essential (Eickers, 2020). In addition, similar to other health care providers, Gender Identity Clinics have suspended face-to-face appointments, put freezes on waitlists, and stopped accepting new referrals (LGBT Foundation, 2020: 20). This is insofar important as these clinics are the only accessible providers of hormones free of charge. In the only empirical study collecting data on the impact of COVID-19 on LGBTQ communities thus far, 61 percent of the respondents stated that they were unable or worried they would not be able to access hormones in the UK due to COVID-19 (LGBT Foundation, 2020: 27). Being unable to access gender affirming care can pose significant mental and physical health challenges for those who are forced to pause their hormone therapy or reschedule long-awaited gender-affirming surgeries.

Infrastructures of mental health for trans* people include accredited counselors and therapists, as well as community organizations and centers, mutual support groups, and social meeting points for LGBTQ people. Access to mental health care poses more challenges for trans* people than for cisgender people, partly due to health practitioners' lack of knowledge of and experience with trans*-related mental health challenges (Ellis et al, 2015). As a consequence, LGBTQ-specific community organizations and services as well as mutual aid groups constitute an essential form of support for trans* people (Eickers, 2020: 27). While experiencing the COVID-19 pandemic is causing increasing levels of stress, depression, anxiety, and insomnia in people across the globe (Mazumder, Chapter Seventeen), these mental health challenges are likely to disproportionately impact trans★ people due to a number of reasons. In addition to a generally higher risk of depression, anxiety, and suicide (Eickers, 2020), social support plays a crucial role for trans★ people's mental health. With the UK lockdown announced in March 2020, trans★ people can no longer access community centers and mutual aid organizations. This means that trans★ people are unable to access these safe places for community building and mutual aid. Such community centers often constitute the only non-private space for trans★ people to build a social life without fear of discrimination or violence, since infrastructures such as public spaces are intimate and deeply gendered in both their impacts and the possibilities they open or foreclose to navigate within them. According to a survey conducted by the LGBT Foundation between April and May 2020, trans★ people found it challenging to access needed specialized mental health support from their communities (LGBT Foundation, 2020: 10). The provision of these support services by LGBTQ organizations is central for the social reproduction of otherwise marginalized individuals. These experiences are further exacerbated by changes in community dynamics.

Community belonging

Research suggests that LGBTQ individuals are more likely to be affected by wider social contexts, including the visibility and cohesiveness of their respective communities (Willging et al, 2006). LGBTQ people in general are more likely to rely on a community or 'chosen family' of close friends and allies for care and support. With the introduction of physical distancing measures and concomitant closing of community centers and queer urban spaces, such as pubs and cafés, social isolation has affected trans★ people in disproportionate ways.

This is likely to be even more prominent for trans* and LGB people, particularly trans* People of Color, aged over 50 years who are more likely to live alone and not own smartphones or computers (LGBT Foundation 2020: 13–14). For trans* individuals, in particular, having a sense of community belongingness is important not only for their well-being but also for their sense of identity (Barr et al, 2016). Not being able to interact and spend time with other LGBTQ people can not only cause feelings of isolation and loss of belonging, but also a disconnect and invisibility of one's identity and the validity of the same. Being seen as the gender a trans* individual identifies is often perceived as essential (McNeil et al, 2012: 71). Losing a sense of self, feeling invisible or invalid, as well as feeling disconnected and not socially embedded can negatively impact trans* individuals' mental health and well-being. Against this backdrop, the support and labor, much of it often invisible, provided by LGBTQ community networks and individuals in queer urban spaces for each other constitutes a form of social reproduction as social infrastructure.

Housing

Not being able to access community support and online therapy sessions can also be due to living in an unsafe environment during lockdown, such as sharing a home with transphobic family or housemates. Having to hide one's gender identity and/or expression can lead to a sense of invalidity and invisibility. In the first two weeks of lockdown between March 23 and April 12, 2020, the LGBT Foundation (2020: 17) recorded a doubled increase in calls about transphobia and trans* individuals feeling unsafe in the places where they were currently staying. Such safety concerns at the level of the home also include experiences of domestic abuse and a higher risk of homelessness, for instance, due to relationship or family breakdown (The Albert Kennedy Trust, 2015).

Trans* people are at a higher risk of becoming homeless or vulnerably housed (Stonewall, 2018) during the COVID-19 lockdown. Reports indicate trans* people, mostly youth, have been forced to live in hostile or abusive situations. In the UK, homelessness charities located in cities such as London and Manchester are experiencing a high volume of LGBTQ youth who are in need of housing assistance. In addition, trans* people are also more at risk of becoming homeless due to precarious labor conditions. This includes jobs in highly affected industries with increased exposure to COVID-19 and higher economic vulnerability, such as gastronomy, retail, and sex work. Being homeless during COVID-19 means transgender and gender non-conforming people are less likely to be able to self-isolate and face difficulties accessing medical care or testing without a fixed address (LGBT Foundation, 2020). Given the high risk of hate crimes against trans* people on the streets, in hospitals, and in shelters, homeless trans* individuals are particularly vulnerable. Against this background, a number of LGBTQ groups both formal and informal, such as the London Bi Pandas, mobilized during lockdown to create and fundraise for emergency funds to provide accessible monetary support to trans* individuals facing homelessness.

Conclusion

Overall, the early phases of the COVID-19 pandemic were marked by a further acceleration of existing inequities for trans* people in cities. With municipal governments already working to narrow their fiscal budget shortfalls and cutting back on social services that benefited economically and socially marginalized people (Forrest, 2020), these developments are likely to continue. At the same time, it is still uncertain how many LGBTQ community spaces will be able to survive the ongoing pandemic, in particular grassroot venues such as queer clubs and bars which prior to the pandemic had already been closing at a high rate since the millennium turn in cities such as London. Given the great importance of urban spaces to provide services that meet the needs of trans* people either residing in sub-/urban locations or traveling outside their rural area to access LGBT services, such developments need to be recorded and further researched.

As a starting point to unpack the unequal experiences of COVID-19 for trans* people, we argue for a relational approach of social infrastructures under austerity. By addressing the interactions, relationships, and institutions that con-figure social infrastructures through health care, community belonging, and housing, we outline how the impacts of the first wave of COVID-19 further diminishes the social reproduction of trans* communities in urban spaces. In early 2021, there remains a dearth of data of the COVID-19 impacts on trans* people in the UK. Given the disproportionate and ongoing impact of COVID-19 on the urban inequities of trans* people, more empirical research is needed to better under-stand and respond to the socially and spatially uneven lived urban experiences of trans* people during the pandemic; the different ways social infrastructures, including forms of social reproduction, have been impacted by and responded to the pandemic; and the specific changes in urban experiences for trans* people along different axes of intersectional inequalities, including ethnicity, class, and age.

References

Amin, A. (2014) 'Lively infrastructure'. *Theory, Culture & Society*, 31(7–8): 137–61.

Barr, S.M., Budge, S.L. and Adelson, J.L. (2016) 'Transgender com-munity belongingness as a mediator between strength of trans-gender identity and well-being'. *Journal of Counselling Psychology*, 63(1): 87–97.

Datta, A. and Ahmed, N. (2020) 'Intimate infrastructures: the rubrics of gendered safety and urban violence in Kerala, India'. *Geoforum*, 110: 67–76.

Doderer, Y.P. (2011) 'LGBTQs in the city, queering urban space'. *International Journal of Urban and Regional Research*, 35(2): 431–6.

Eickers, G. (2020) 'COVID-19 and trans healthcare: yes, global pandemics are (also) a trans rights issue'. *Gender Forum, Special Issue: Gender in Crisis: Covid-19 and Its Impact*, 19–34.

Ellis, S., Bailey, L. and McNeil, J. (2015) 'Trans people's experiences of mental health and gender identity services: a UK study'. *Journal of Gay & Lesbian Mental Health*, 19(1): 1–17.

Forrest, A. (2020) 'Coronavirus: UK towns and cities warn of potential bankruptcy due to the pandemic'. *The Independent*. www.independent.co.uk/news/uk/politics/coronavirus-uk-cities-bankruptcy-emergency-funding-a9584986.html

Gieseking, J. (2015) 'Urban margins on the move: rethinking LGBTQ inclusion by queering the place of the gayborhood'. *Berliner Blätter – Ethnographische und ethnologische Beiträge*, 68: 43–5.

Hall, S.M. (2015) 'Everyday ethics of consumption in the austere city'. *Geography Compass*, 9: 140–51.

Hall, S.M. (2020) 'Social reproduction as social infrastructure'. *Soundings: A journal of Politics and Culture*, 76: 82–94.

Hardy, S.J. and Chakraborti, N. (2015) *LGB&T hate crime reporting: identifying barriers and solutions*. Research report. Leicester: University of Leicester.

Kattari, S.K., Whitfield, D.L., DeChants, J. and Alvarez, A.R.G. (2016) *Barriers to health faced by transgender and non-binary black and minority ethnic people*. A Race Equality Foundation Briefing Paper. www.raceequalityfoundation.org.uk/wp-content/uploads/2018/02/Better-Health-41-Trans-NB-final.pdf

LGBT Foundation (2020) *Hidden figures: the impact of the COVID-19 pandemic on LGBT communities in the UK*, 3rd edition. https://s3-eu-west-1.amazonaws.com/lgbt-website-media/Files/7a01b983-b54b-4dd3-84b2-0f2ecd72be52/Hidden%2520Figures-%2520The%2520Impact%2520of%2520the%2520Covid-19%2520Pandemic%2520on%2520LGBT%2520Communities.pdf

McNeil, J., Bailey, L. and Ellis, S., Morton, J. and Regan, M. (2012) *Trans mental health and emotional wellbeing study, 1–94.* Retrieved from: www.gires.org.uk/wp-content/uploads/2014/08/trans_mh_study.pdf

Siemiatycki, M., Enright, T. and Valverde, M. (2020) 'The gendered production of infrastructure'. *Progress in Human Geography,* 44(2): 297–314.

Simone, A. (2004) 'People as infrastructure: intersecting fragments in Johannesburg'. *Public Culture,* 16(3): 407–29.

Stonewall (2018) *LGBT in Britain: Trans report, 1–23.* www.stonewall.org.uk/system/files/lgbt_in_britain_-_trans_report_final.pdf

The Albert Kennedy Trust (2015) *LGBT youth homelessness: a UK national scoping of cause, prevalence, response & outcome.* www.akt.org.uk/research

Willging, C.E., Salvador, M. and Kano, M. (2006) 'Unequal treatment: mental health care for sexual and gender minority groups in a rural state'. *Psychiatric Services,* 57(6): 867–70.

Wilson, A. (2016) 'The infrastructure of intimacy'. *Signs: Journal of Women in Culture and Society,* 41(2): 247–80.

TWENTY-ONE

COVID-19 and Blind Spaces: Responding to Digital (In)Accessibility and Social Isolation During Lockdown for Blind, Deafblind, Low Vision, and Vision Impaired Persons in Aotearoa New Zealand

Rebekah Graham, Bridgette Masters-Awatere,
Chrissie Cowan, Amanda Stevens, and Rose Wilkinson

In response to increasing confirmed cases of COVID-19, the resident population of Aotearoa New Zealand entered a seven-week lockdown at midnight on March 25, 2020. The first five weeks were at level 4, with the population instructed to remain in their homes and associate only with those in their immediate household. All public gatherings were banned, non-essential businesses required to close public-facing services, domestic travel severely curtailed, and the border closed to all non-citizens. Official sources of information were daily 1pm briefings by the Prime Minister and the Director General of Health. These were broadcast live via radio, television, news websites, and social media. There was also a dedicated COVID-19 information website.[1] The requirement to stay at home saw increased numbers of people working from home and increased use of video conferencing software (for example Zoom) as a mechanism for 'meeting with' colleagues, family, and friends. In this manner, digital and associated technologies extended the interpersonal space of the home beyond the physical confines of the domestic dwelling, drawing people together in digital spaces. Digital technologies integrated the previously separated workspace into the home environment allowing work colleagues to 'see into' personal spaces (see Hubbard, Volume 2; van Melik et al, Volume 3). This blurring of work and home shifted thinking about work contexts. Overall, the combination of lockdown, daily briefings, and increased digital connectivity contributed to a sense of shared experience across the country. However, these shared experiences were not equally available across the citizenry, with the COVID-19 pandemic exacerbating existing inequities.

Contemporary digital spaces inhabited during lockdown prioritized the needs of the fully able citizenry. Consequently, inherited power structures and hierarchies were digitally (re)produced (Lefebvre, 1991). Everyday space is typically designed by and for non-disabled people (Chouinard et al, 2010). Additionally, disabled people are marginalized from everyday social, economic, and political processes and spaces (Milner and Kelly, 2009). As a result, disabled persons are prevented from full participation as active and engaged citizens by abled persons in positions of decision-making power. In understanding the ways in which digital space(s) were (re)produced for blind, deafblind, low vision and vision impaired (BLV) persons during COVID-19 lockdown we make visible how contemporary urban society perpetuates historical processes of exclusion.

Aotearoa New Zealand's founding document, Te Tiriti o Waitangi,[2] is an agreement between Māori (Indigenous people of Aotearoa) and the Crown to reside together as equal partners. To that end, our chapter brings together Māori (Bridgette Masters-Awatere, Chrissie Cowan) and non-Māori authors (Rebekah Graham, Amanda Stevens, Rose Wilkinson) in critically examining the experiences of BLV persons during the COVID-19 lockdown. In considering these experiences we also acknowledge the value of working together as academics (Graham, Masters-Awatere) and disability advocates (Cowan, Stevens, Wilkinson). Aotearoa New Zealand is also a signatory to the United Nations Convention on the Rights of Persons with Disabilities (CRPD) and to the United Nations Declaration on the Rights of Indigenous Peoples (UNDRIP). Despite a stated commitment to disabled persons and to Māori, economic and accessibility inequities for both groups remain entrenched. Historical experiences by persons with disabilities are of being marginalized from economic opportunities and excluded from societal participation (Johnson, 2020). Disabled persons and Māori are disproportionately represented in Aotearoa New Zealand's disparity statistics (Hickey, 2020; Johnson, 2020), and digital access is no exception. Twenty-nine percent of New Zealanders with disabilities do not have internet access (Grimes and White, 2019). Māori are also over-represented in digital exclusion statistics, with factors such as poverty, health, education, and social needs that disadvantage Māori generally having a direct correlation to the accessibility of digital spaces (Citizens Advice Bureaux (CAB), 2020). Despite government awareness of these inequities, progress towards ensuring inclusivity in digital spaces has been slow-moving.

Digital exclusion (those who have limited or no access to or won't or can't use digital technology) occurs along existing lines of inequitable access to resources and insufficient funding (Grimes and White, 2019); the biggest barrier to digital access is poverty (CAB, 2020). Prior to the pandemic, people with a range of disabilities engaged with publicly funded services such as Citizens Advice Bureaux and local libraries to access information via the internet and navigate online spaces. It was not uncommon for low-income and older BLV persons to utilize internet services via their local library, which typically offers free internet access alongside familiar text-to-speech software for use with digital technologies. With such services closed due to the nationwide lockdown, BLV persons found themselves disconnected and locked out of digital spaces (see also Turman et al, Volume 2; Corble and van Melik, Volume 3).

Digital exclusion also occurs when websites are inaccessible. During Aotearoa New Zealand's first[3] experience of COVID-19 lockdown, digital sites such as social media and websites were key spaces for the dissemination of health information. While Aotearoa New Zealand has made legislative efforts with accessibility (for example Office of the Minister of State Services, 2003; Office of the Minister for Disability Issues, 2020), the initial response to COVID-19 did not reflect this progress. The initial dedicated COVID-19 website did not meet the government's web guidelines for minimum requirements for government websites (as outlined in the aforementioned 2003 cabinet paper) with regard to accessible design and content. This oversight resulted in BLV persons who did have digital technologies and internet access within the domestic space of their home being unable to access timely and up-to-date information regarding COVID-19. This was particularly problematic in the context of a deadly global pandemic where health information was fast-paced and constantly changing. Despite legal protections and recognized rights as per Article 9 of the CRPD,[4] the (re)production of inequities in digital spaces during a rapidly shifting environment re-marginalized and excluded BLV persons.

During the COVID-19 lockdown, digital spaces became key sites for engaging in societal interactions, retaining social support systems, and extending the life-space (Lewin, 2013). Life-spaces stretch through time and space and are ordered by the strength of the relationship, not the physical distance (Lewin, 2013). Life-space connections became even more important during a nationwide lockdown constraining people to the domestic space of the home and severely curtailing in-person interactions. The life-space of BLV persons and a corresponding sense of agency, independence, and dignity was impacted by the shift to digital spaces for social interactions. For example, a BLV person may have digital technology and internet access but requires a sighted family member or support worker to guide them through first-time use of new websites and applications. Without in-person support, navigating first-time use of a video conferencing tool becomes next to impossible. In this way, for BLV persons left without necessary supports, the relational space(s) they inhabited were spatially and temporally reduced. This in turn impacted on their sense of agency, independence, and dignity.

In response to increased digital exclusion at a time of increased digital reliance, BLV organizations (such as those represented in the authorship of this chapter) advocated with government ministries and provided financial and practical assistance to BLV persons. Challenging reproductions of power and exclusion required sustained effort and creative thinking at a time of great stress. For example, BLV organizations arranged to print and post hard copies of COVID-19-related information in Braille and Large Print formats, as well as audio CDs. Doing so necessitated creative interpretations of lock-down regulations and subverting the newly imposed social norms. BLV organizations also strengthened existing relational networks via familiar technologies (for example telephone) in order to mitigate experiences of exclusion. Being able to maintain and sustain a sense of connection with others is vital to fostering a sense of belonging. BLV persons who were embedded within existing communities and whose communities were able to sustain social interactions via telephone and postal services found the lockdown was less corrosive to their sense of belonging. However, for BLV persons without access to their usual supports, the experiences of lockdown brought new and increasing levels of social isolation. This contributed to a reduced a sense of belonging and left people feeling 'forgotten' by wider society.

In this next section we aim to make visible the narratives and experiences of BLV Māori (kāpō Māori). Māori move in and through a range of subjectivities at different times and in different places (Simmonds, 2011). Being Māori and being disabled positions kāpō Māori in complex and tricky spaces that require careful negotiation. This includes embodied geographies of place and space that are localized and place specific (Simmonds, 2011), as well as constructions of disability that are not a separate identity but rather a natural consequence of life itself (Hickey, 2020). As such, the life-spaces of kāpō Māori are textured with past and future relational connections as well as cultural understandings of what it means to be Māori here and now.

As a group, Māori have a long history of decision-making that prioritizes the health and well-being of their people (Graham and Masters-Awatere, 2020). Prior to the COVID-19 lockdown, digital spaces were drawn on to support well-being of whānau (family), with whānau members interacting online to maintain relational links and uphold shared values (Keegan and Sciascia, 2018). During lockdown, the value of whānau well-being came to the fore, with kāpō Māori remaining connected to one another through acts of caring and support. This included mundane activities such as supermarket shopping and telephone calls, through to the organizing of care packages and health checks. These acts reduced a sense of isolation, increased a sense of care and connection, and reinforced the shared values and identities associated with being Māori (Simmonds, 2011).

Throughout the pandemic iwi (Māori tribal) leaders continually made decisions that had the health and well-being of their people at the center, such as the decision to close roads into Māori communities. Despite this and stated commitments to Te Tiriti and UNDRIP, the Aotearoa New Zealand government struggled to trust iwi leaders to determine culturally appropriate practice during lockdown. This was evident in government officials specifically naming marae (Māori meeting ground) as a space where the police could enact 'no-knock order beaches' during the lockdown period. That is, marae were singled out as spaces that agents of the Crown could enter without asking and without following the usual cultural protocols. The absence of shared decision-making processes was also exemplified in decisions regarding tangihanga (Māori funeral rituals) which saw a primarily non-Māori decision-making team imposing new rules onto tangihanga during lockdown.

Tangihanga as a cultural practice reflects ongoing change as values and practical realities change across generations (Nikora et al, 2012). Recent adaptions have seen increased use of digital technologies to meet cultural needs of the Māori diaspora (O'Carroll, 2015). Instead of lockdown changes to tangihanga practices being determined in conjunction with iwi leaders and kaumātua (elders), the dominant colonial values and ideological parameters of the Crown were imposed on Māori. This directly impacted on kāpō Māori kaumātua. One kāpō Māori kaumātua, who would usually speak on the marae paepae (orators' bench) to farewell and honor a loved one during tangihanga, was deeply distressed at being locked out of determining how to best adjust his cultural practice to meet the needs of his bereaved whānau. The role of guiding the bereavement for whānau is a core part of identity as a kaumātua and reflects a shared responsibility to represent and connect the past with the present. Being unable to fulfill this core role resulted in feelings of grief and a sense of being 'cut off' from vital cultural spaces. Compounding these feelings was the imposition of government rule over-riding Māori self-determination, resulting in non-Māori dictating to Māori how they enacted their own cultural practices. Doing so reproduced historical power relationships and cultural memories of distrust, causing harm and negatively impacting on a sense of agency over one's own cultural spaces and practices.

In reflecting on our combined experiences and observations, we note improvements by government departments in providing information in an accessible format in a timelier manner (in September 2020, the wait time was three working days). We also note increased commitment to partnership with Māori, such as the implementation of an Iwi Chairs Forum for COVID-19-related matters. Such examples give us hope that Aotearoa New Zealand, as a government and as a society, is committed to improving inclusivity and accessibility. However, poverty-related exclusion remains. Low-income households continue to have reduced access to digital technologies and appropriate protective equipment, such as face masks (which bring their own challenges for disabled persons). The general public, while well-meaning, still struggle to consider the needs of disabled persons. For example, despite clear requests to place NZ COVID-19 Tracer QR code posters[5] 'on the left-hand side of your front window or entrance, with the top approximately 130cm from the ground', posters were located at inaccessible heights for wheelchair users, and inconsistently placed with regard to height and location, making them difficult for BLV persons to locate and use.

As we have documented in our chapter, decision-making processes remain textured with implicit bias, racism, and ableism. The complexities and nuances of issues such as website access and imposed tangihanga rules were brushed aside and/or rendered invisible. There is potential societal risk if we continue to exclude disabled persons and Māori from decision-making spaces. We need a systems shift. We must primarily design around the needs of disabled and marginalized persons, rather than being designed for and by people who are fully able, healthy, and with access to economic resources.

Notes

1   www.covid19.govt.nz
2   There are two versions: one in English (the Treaty of Waitangi) and one in te reo Māori (Te Tiriti of Waitangi). Throughout this chapter we refer to Te Tiriti, the version written in te reo Māori.
3   By April 2021, the Auckland metropolis and greater Auckland region (with a combined population of 1.71 million) had experienced an additional three instances of Level 3 restrictions.
4   Full text of Article 9 – Accessibility of the UNCRPD can be found at www.un.org/development/desa/disabilities/convention-on-the-rights-of-persons-with-disabilities/article-9-accessibility.html
5   See www.health.govt.nz/our-work/diseases-and-conditions/covid-19-novel-coronavirus/covid-19-resources-and-tools/nz-covid-tracer-app/nz-covid-tracer-qr-codes

References

Chouinard, V., Hall, E. and Wilton, R. (2010) *Towards Enabling Geographies: 'Disabled' Bodies and Minds in Society and Space*. Surrey, UK: Ashgate.

Citizens Advice Bureaux (CAB) (2020) *Face to face with digital exclusion*. Wellington, NZ. www.cab.org.nz/assets/Documents/Face-to-Face-with-Digital-Exclusion-/9c5f26012e/Face-to-face-with-Digital-Exclusion.pdf

Graham, R. and Masters-Awatere, B. (2020) 'Experiences of Māori of Aotearoa New Zealand's public health system: a systematic review of two decades of published qualitative research'. *Australian and New Zealand Journal of Public Health*, 44(3): 193–200.

Grimes, A. and White, D. (2019) *Digital inclusion and wellbeing in New Zealand*. Motu Working Paper 19–17. Motu Economic and Public Policy Research. Wellington, NZ: DIA.

Hickey, H. (2020) 'A personal reflection on indigeneity, colonisation and the CRPD', in E.J. Kakoullis and K. Johnson (eds) *Recognising Human Rights in Different Cultural Contexts*. Singapore: Palgrave Macmillan, pp 79–93.

Johnson, K. (2020) 'Recognising cultural diversity: implications for persons with disabilities', in E.J. Kakoullis and K. Johnson (eds) *Recognising Human Rights in Different Cultural Contexts*. Singapore: Palgrave Macmillan, pp 63–78.

Keegan, T.T. and Sciascia, A. (2018) 'Hangarau mete Maori: Maori and technology', in M. Reilly, S. Duncan, G. Leoni, L. Paterson, L. Carter, M. Rātima and P. Rewi (eds) *Te Kōparapara: An Introduction to the Māori World*. Auckland, NZ: Auckland University Press, pp 359–71.

Lefebvre, H. (1991) *The Production of Space*. Malden, MA: Blackwell.

Lewin, K. (2013) *Principles of Topological Psychology*. Redditch, UK: Read Books (original work published 1936).

Milner, P. and Kelly, B. (2009) 'Community participation and inclusion: people with disabilities defining their place'. *Disability & Society*, 24(1): 47–62.

Nikora, L.W., Masters-Awatere, B. and te Awekotuku, N. (2012) 'Final arrangements following death: Maori Indigenous decision-making and tangi'. *Journal of Community & Applied Social Psychology*, 22(5): 400–13.

O'Carroll, A.D. (2015) 'Virtual tangihanga, virtual tikanga: investigating the potential and pitfalls of virtualising Māori cultural practice'. *The Canadian Journal of Native Studies*, 35(2): 183–206.

Office of the Minister for Disability Issues (2020) *Accelerating progress towards accessibility in New Zealand*. www.msd.govt.nz/documents/about-msd-and-our-work/publications-resources/information-releases/cabinet-paper-on-accelerating-accessibility.pdf

Office of the Minister of State Services (2003) *Cabinet paper: New Zealand government web guidelines*. www.digital.govt.nz/standards-and-guidance/nz-government-web-standards/new-zealand-government-web-guidelines-cabinet-paper-and-minute/cabinet-paper-new-zealand-government-web-guidelines/

Simmonds, N. (2011) 'Mana wāhine: decolonising politics'. *Women's Studies Journal*, 25(2): 11–25.

TWENTY-TWO

Conclusion

Brian Doucet, Rianne van Melik, and Pierre Filion

On October 28, 2020, Canada's Chief Medical Officer of Health, Dr Theresa Tam, stated that the pandemic was exposing existing inequalities in Canada. In a television address, she said that:

> 'The impacts of COVID-19 in this country have been worsened by systems that stigmatize populations through racism, ageism, sexism, and others, who have been marginalized through structural or social factors such as homelessness ... Differences [in infection rates] are not random, but all along the lines of populations that have historically experienced health and social inequities ... The impacts have been worse for some groups such as seniors, workers who provide essential services, such as those in health care or agriculture, racialized populations, people living with disabilities, and women. The virus didn't create new inequities in our society; it exposed them and underscored the impact of our social policies on our health status'.[1]

While this may have been a revelation for some people, for the contributors to this volume, and the others in this series, such a direct and unequivocal statement was not surprising.

Such insights are also nothing new to those with lived experiences of these inequalities and injustices. Throughout the four volumes, one of our aims has been to include chapters that amplify these voices by meaningfully, respectfully, and ethically engaging with marginalized communities in order to center their experiences within planning, policy, and political debates about the impact of the pandemic and, importantly, how to respond to it. The findings, analysis, and reflection found throughout this series of books must be a reminder to planners and policy makers that the divisions, inequities, and injustices rendered visible during the COVID-19 pandemic long predate the virus. As a result, any meaningful policies to address them must primarily focus on the structural forces that produce unequal cities and societies.

The chapters in this volume prompt us to ask two important questions. First, does the pandemic require us to think of new ideas or solutions? Or phrased another way, can the challenges of the pandemic be addressed by implementing policies that scholars, advocates, and practitioners have been calling for for many years? Is it a question of new ideas, or changing priorities? Related to this, the second question we must ask is this: what social, economic, planning, and political factors need to change in order to build more equitable cities? Finally, we need to ask what role, if any, has the pandemic played in altering these factors?

With these questions in mind, we offer two critical reflections that can help guide and inform urban debates. First, it is important to stress that many of the inequalities that have been rendered visible during the pandemic will not simply abate once it is over. The stark differences and inequalities we are witnessing during the pandemic are built on layers of injustice that are years, decades, and even centuries in the making. The pandemic has amplified these economic, social, spatial, and racial divisions in often catastrophic ways. This is why calls for a return to the normality of the pre-pandemic period are highly problematic.

Compounding these pre-existing inequalities are many of the planning and policy measures rapidly implemented to deal with immediate challenges of the pandemic. These have often been designed to be temporary, and do not address structural or systemic inequalities (Parsell et al, 2020; Vilenica et al, 2020). As explored further in Volume 2, they reinforce, rather than challenge pre-existing inequities and power relations. For example, in 2020, planning departments in cities around the world expedited applications for sidewalk patios in order to provide outdoor dining opportunities for established businesses and corporate chains. Yet, as Amina Yasin and Daniella Ferguson (2021) note, marginalized groups who also use those same sidewalks, such as unsheltered individuals, or street vendors selling food (who are often from racialized communities), have seen very little to address their long-standing challenges, and very little planning support to assist with their livelihoods. Planning responses to the immediate challenges of the pandemic have privileged some groups while ignoring others.

Therefore, instead of speculating about what cities will be like in future, our second point of reflection examines *how* to build a more equitable post-pandemic urban future by focusing on the question of *who* is included in the planning, policy, and political conversations that will determine the future of cities? Who is excluded from them? Whose voices are represented at the decision-making table? Who is absent? Who decides which voices are present? Who is there to tick a box, and who are the ones actually making the decisions? These are difficult questions that require more than inviting people to an open house or participating in a community consultation process. While built form, urban design, land use, and architecture are all important factors that shape our different experiences of urban life, many chapters in this volume emphasize how marginalized individuals and communities have very little *power* over the decisions that shape urban space. As Graham et al (Chapter Twenty-One) noted: 'decision-making processes remain textured with implicit bias, racism, and ableism'.

This volume has highlighted how, for many, even the most basic opportunities to contribute to the decision-making process are absent. The authors of Chapter Nineteen on experiences of older adults in the Netherlands state that: 'we mainly talk *about* and decide *for* older adults, *instead* of with them'. Domestic workers in the US (Chapter Four), *hustlers* in Jamaica (Chapter Five), migrants in Dhaka (Chapter Thirteen), Singapore (Chapter Sixteen), and Kuala Lumpur (Chapter Fourteen), Rohingya refugees living in Bangladesh (Chapter Fifteen), and many others have very little power over the decisions that shape their lives, and therefore rely on the decisions made by others who rarely have their interests in mind. When discussing the plight of migrant workers in Dubai, Abdellatif Qamhaieh (Chapter Three) noted that while they constitute a sizable percentage of the city's population, they are kept silent in important conversations about the city, explaining that: 'they provide valuable services to the community, without which it will not function. Still they remain casual observers, and are never really expected to belong or participate'.

Planning is about power, and as Tamika Butler (2020), an urban planner, activist, and public speaker based in Los Angeles reminds us, to achieve equitable cities, those with power will need to relinquish some of it in order that other, currently marginalized groups, can have more. This is the big challenge facing cities in the post-pandemic period. These power relations also constitute an important element of continuity between the pandemic and pre-pandemic periods; while much has changed since the arrival of COVID-19, more than a year into the pandemic, the power relations that govern cities and urban space have shifted very little. On the surface, the pandemic appears to have changed everything about urban life. However, as the chapters within this volume have demonstrated, it is also clear that political economies governing planning and policy making in cities around the world have remained largely static, although as Dilworth and Weaver (Chapter Eighteen) note, the pandemic has opened up the door for some, once radical ideas, to enter mainstream conversations.

Therefore, to create a more equitable post-pandemic future, listening to marginalized communities and using positions of privilege to amplify their voices is only the first, albeit important step, that can start shifting conversations and debates. Ultimately, however, the power relations which govern cities and urban space will need to fundamentally shift if the post-pandemic city is going to be a more equitable, or socially just one.

Note

[1] www.cbc.ca/player/play/1812702787589

References

Butler, T. (2020) *LiveMove Speaker Series: The Intersection of Racism and Transportation,* October 31. www.tamikabutler.com/media/2020/10/31/livemove-speaker-series-the-intersection-of-racism-and-transportation

Parsell, C., Clarke, A. and Kuskoff, E. (2020) 'Understanding responses to homelessness during COVID-19: an examination of Australia'. *Housing Studies*, 1–14. https://doi.org/10.1080/02673037.2020.1829564

Vilenica, A., McElroy, E., Ferreri, M., Fernández Arrigoitia, M., García-Lamarca, M. and Lancione, M. (2020) 'COVID-19 and housing struggles: the (re) makings of austerity, disaster capitalism, and the no return to normal'. *Radical Housing Journal*, 2(1): 9–28.

Yasin, A. and Ferguson, D. (2021) 'Pandemic patios and "flat-white" urbanism'. *Plan Canada*, 60(4): 21–6.

Index

References to endnotes show both the page number and the note number (for example, 231n3).

Printed and bound by CPI Group (UK) Ltd, Croydon, CR0 4YY

07/07/2026

14916219-0002